THE 7 PRINCIPLES OF FAT BURNING

THE 7 PRINCIPLES OF FAT BURNING

Get healthy, lose weight and keep it off!

ERIC BERG, DC

ACTION PUBLISHING | LOS ANGELES

Limit of Liability/Disclaimer of Warranty

This book is not intended as a substitute for the medical recommendations of physicians or other healthcare providers. Rather, it is intended to offer information for educational purposes and to help the reader cooperate with physicians and health professionals in a joint quest for optimum health.

The information discussed in this book—including any dietary and other substances and materials, products, equipment or devices—has not undergone evaluation and testing by the U.S. Food and Drug Administration or similar agency of any other country and is not intended to diagnose, treat, prevent, mitigate or cure any disease. Please consult with a physician or other healthcare professional before utilizing any of the information from this book. The reader and user should treat this information as a general guide and not as the ultimate source of information, as it is based on the opinion and sole experience of Eric Berg, DC. The information reported as results achieved by particular individuals should not be considered as typical, and the reader or user should not believe that the reader or user might achieve the same results. The advice and strategies contained herein may not be suitable for your situation. You should consult with a professional where appropriate.

While the publisher and the author have used their best efforts in preparing this book, they make no representations or warranties with respect to the accuracy or completeness of the contents of this book and specifically disclaim any implied warranties of merchantability or fitness for a particular purpose. No warranty may be created or extended by sales representatives or written sales materials. Neither the publisher nor the author is responsible for any goods and/or services referred to in this book, and both expressly disclaim all liability in connection with the fulfillment of orders for any such goods and/or services or for any damages, loss or expense to person or property arising out of or relating to them. Neither the publisher nor the author shall be liable for any loss of profit or any other commercial damages, including but not limited to special, incidental or consequential damages.

Regular exercise and proper nutrition are essential for achieving your weight-loss goal.

Illustrations by Allen Harris at www.livinglightning.com

ISBN-10: 1-888045-55-8
ISBN-13: 978-1-888045-55-0

Printed in the United States of America

10 9 8 7 6 5 4 3 2

Action Publishing, LLC
P.O. Box 391
Glendale, CA 91209
www.actionpublishing.com

For more health information from Dr. Berg, visit www.bergdiets.com.

To my beautiful wife, Karen,
and my fantastic children,
Jordan, Allison and Ian,
for putting up with my being
so often in the "cave" office,
behind the computer screen.

Contents

Charts

1

Missing Link — the Educational Step

Have you ever felt that it shouldn't be so hard or take so much effort to lose even a little bit of weight? Well, the last thing you need is another diet! If you are simply told what to eat and it doesn't work for you, you'll chalk up a loss and go on to the next diet, creating further losses, and then think there is a problem with you, that you have poor willpower (an inability to stick with something).

Working with thousands of individuals has led me to believe that people really do *not* have a problem with willpower—they simply have never been taught the right way to lose weight. No one is going to stick with a program that's not working. But if you do the correct thing and *you know how to do it*, it *will* work and you will stick with it.

In my clinic, I have found that the missing link is an educational step. Once a person has the background and understanding of HOW fat is burned and HOW health is created, they succeed. But if you simply tell them what to do, you've done nothing for them of any lasting value.

There are so many weight loss books out there that say, "Scientific studies have shown . . . " or "Everyone knows . . . " or "Experts say . . . " That type of approach is very far from conveying understanding.

This book is different.

I want to help you solve a big problem—stubborn weight. To do that, we must first make sure we have identified the *correct* problem. Many people are attempting to fix the wrong problem: their weight (which is actually the symptom). You also need to know what controls metabolism—hormones—because you are going to use these hormones to work for you instead of against you. Hormones are chemical messages produced by glands. You have six fat-burning and three fat-making hormones, and each is triggered by different things. Might it not be a good idea to know *what* these are and *how* to trigger them?

The 7 Principles of Fat Burning is not necessarily for people who can lose weight easily; it is for those who have a very stubborn metabolism. *The 7 Principles of Fat Burning* gives you the most effective leverage over weight loss because it addresses the very things that control weight loss—fat-burning hormones. To my knowledge, no other book in existence gives you an easy-to-understand summary of how to use food and activities to trigger all of your fat-burning hormones. Most people don't even know these exist, let alone how to get them to work.

Fat is not a cushion or insulation, as many people think, but is a store of reserve energy, and I'm about to show you how to get your body to tap into and run on this energy. Most people are running their bodies on sugar fuel and rarely use fat fuel, yet right now you already have within your own body everything you need in order to tap into your fat reserves.

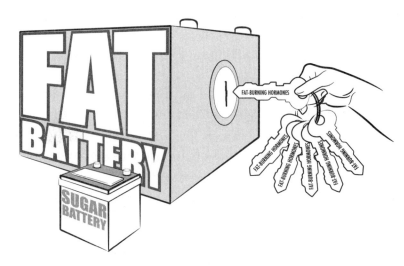

You are going to be triggering not just one hormone but *all* six key hormones to create maximum fat-burning effects. As a result, you not only

WILL lose major weight but will get extremely healthy at the same time. The nice thing is that some of these hormones are antiaging as well.

Different bodies need different solutions. I have found that most people fall into four different types and need different variations of food (especially protein) and exercise. In chapter 4, you'll be taking a quiz to find out which body type you have. Once you start the eating plan, you'll soon find out what your body responds to best in order to lose the most weight possible in the shortest period of time with the least effort.

What you might not have realized is that your own hormones have been working against you, making you fat and distorting your body's shape. Instead of giving you the same old same old, I'm going to help you find out which hormone or gland is responsible for your body type and guide you to the best program to fix the problem.

You will not be allowed to get hungry, cut calories, starve yourself or skip a meal. You will be eating nutrient-dense foods, which will knock out cravings for sweets, breads, salty snacks and chocolate and keep you satisfied.

For the first two weeks you will be on the Liver Enhancement Plan, which will prepare you for better fat burning later on. Did you realize that all your fat-burning hormones work through your liver? So, by giving it a good cleaning, things will work faster and more easily for you. The liver needs lots of raw and steamed vegetables, some fruits, especially apples, raw nuts and a very special cranberry drink, which you will be using to speed up the process. This is where you'll start noticing your clothes are looser, particularly around your midsection.

After completing this step, you will start increasing proteins until you get the right amount for your body. You will then continue this combination of foods until you achieve your ideal health and weight. The secret is to specifically address your main glandular weakness as opposed to the shotgun treat-everything approach. Each fat-burning hormone has different triggers and you are going to use them ALL.

This is a lifestyle change, not just a diet you do to lose weight and then go back to junk foods. It has been our experience that as people increase their health, their bodies no longer desire refined sweet foods but crave nutrient-dense whole foods.

Anyone can lose weight on just about any diet. The most unique and exciting thing about this program is that you will be able to keep the weight off because you are correcting the cause. With this program, you will be stabilizing the glands and hormones that have been responsible for making you fat in the first place. If you simply do what everyone else is doing — losing the weight without fixing the cause of the problem — the weight will just come right back. Your primary goal needs to be getting your weakest gland healthy so that you can stay permanently at your ideal weight.

The absolute maximum fat a person can burn per week is two pounds. However, water weight can come off at two to five pounds per day in some cases. In one extreme case, I had a patient eliminate a full bladder of fluid 12 times within a 24-hour period. So, how much water weight or fat weight you have will determine how quickly you will lose the weight. But the problem you've been running into is that your own hormone system has been blocked, preventing your body from burning fat and from losing water weight. Our goal is to fix this problem and keep you in fat-burning mode throughout this entire process.

Your energy will be significantly increased and your sleep will become much sounder and deeper; your digestion will improve and your nails, skin and hair will also be in better condition, because hormones control these body activities and characteristics. Many of my patients have lowered cholesterol and blood pressure on this program as well.

Through a study of this book you will identify your own body type and learn some fascinating things about how your body works and how it stops working, especially in regard to fat burning. The idea is to teach you how to look beyond diets and exercise and instead use hormone triggers from foods and exercise. This way you will never have to depend on a program but will be in full control of your own weight and health. Nobody will have to tell you what to eat at a social gathering or a restaurant because you yourself will be able to tell the difference between what causes fat and what burns fat.

We are talking about the thing that you live in — your body — and since you do live inside it, it might be of benefit to understand the owner's manual.

2

The 7 Principles of Fat Burning

Many people have been trying to lose weight with various diet and exercise programs. Everywhere you look you see another diet popping up — cabbage soup, cookie, peanut butter, grapefruit, high-protein, etc. I want you to take another route. I want you to understand what's behind a stubborn and resistant metabolism before you jump into the solution.

The clinic at my northern Virginia Health & Wellness Center has been an excellent testing ground, working with thousands of different types of patients, using diet, exercise and nutrition. The center provides a variety of health modalities, from counseling on nutrition and healthy eating to my Acupressure Stress Elimination Technique (ASET). Any increase in stress triggers the adrenal hormone cortisol, which blocks fat burning. This technique deals with reducing body stress.*

The Purpose of Food

A main confusion many people have is with the very definition of *food* and its purpose. They think of it as "something you eat to get pleasure, to reward and treat yourself with." But in no dictionary could I find this definition. Check out the following definition from the *Macmillan Dictionary*:

---

* For more information, see the glossary, page 283, and the resources section, page 313.

Food *n.* that which is eaten to sustain life, provide energy, and promote the growth and repair of tissues; nourishment [Old English *fōda*, "nourishment"]

According to this definition, a lot of people are living on something other than food. Let me tell you what I do when I am shopping at the grocery store or eating at a restaurant. I ask myself several questions: Is this an imitation of food or a man-made food-like substance? Will this substance ADD more life, more health, and will it nourish and repair my tissues, or will it reduce my health?

The question now becomes, how do we classify or know which foods are really foods and which are nonfoods? What substances are essential to life? What substances can we not live without? What is the body made out of, which if missing will create illness?

The vital substances necessary to the body are referred to as "essential"—as in *essential amino acids* and *essential fatty acids. Essential* means "cannot be made by the body and MUST come from the diet." Amino acids, for example, are the building blocks that make our hair, nails, eyes, muscles, joints, etc. Fatty acids make up the outer and inner structures of our cells, not to mention our brains, nerves and hormones.

There are many nutrients that if missing from the body will cause disease. These essential raw materials must also include vitamins and minerals. And enzymes must be added to this list because consuming foods that are void of enzymes can create degenerative diseases. Enzymes are the things that do the work of the body, similar to assembly workers in a factory.

Foodstuffs that contain all of these nutrients are more *food* than those that leave out these factors or contain them but in a destroyed or altered form, as happens when food is cooked, pasteurized, processed or roasted. Simply stated, foods containing all these factors—amino acids, fatty acids, vitamins, minerals and enzymes—and in an optimum balance would create the most health. This is why isolated food factors such as those in protein shakes (isolated soy protein), synthetic vitamins (petroleum derivatives), refined sugars and carbohydrates (which have to be enriched with synthetic vitamins because they are depleted) are more *nonfoods* than anything else. So, we have a scale from healing foods to illness-creating nonfoods. This book is about consuming foods that naturally contain all five building blocks. With our computerized program called the Fat-Burning-Tracker Coach, we are able to rate a person's diet as to how closely it fits the definition of *food* and how much health they are creating.*

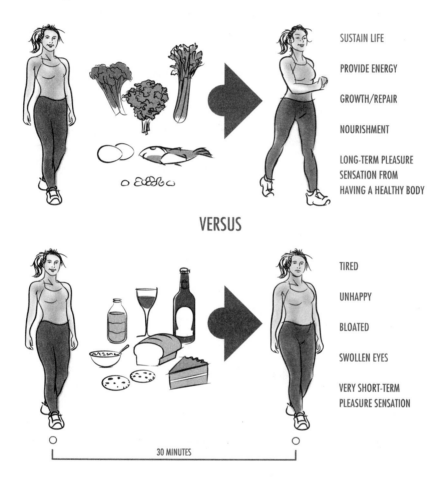

VERSUS

SUSTAIN LIFE

PROVIDE ENERGY

GROWTH/REPAIR

NOURISHMENT

LONG-TERM PLEASURE
SENSATION FROM
HAVING A HEALTHY BODY

TIRED

UNHAPPY

BLOATED

SWOLLEN EYES

VERY SHORT-TERM
PLEASURE SENSATION

30 MINUTES

food *n.* that which is eaten to sustain life, provide energy, and promote the growth and repair of tissues [Old English *fōda*, "nourishment"]

The word *diet* also has an interesting derivation.

Diet *n.* a regulated course of food and drink to promote health or for weight control — *v.i.* to eat according to prescribed rules [Old French *diète*, from Latin *diaeta*, **"way of living"**]

---

* See chapter 3, pages 34–35.

Diet stems from the word meaning "a way of living"—which is an interesting new viewpoint compared to the older idea of "something people do to deprive and starve themselves."

By understanding and then applying this broader concept of eating and living to create health as you go through this program, you WILL end up with the byproduct of a slim, healthy body.

The following are the seven key principles on which our program is based.

Principle #1

There Are Four Different Body Shapes, Each Influenced by Hormones

You might have heard of pear and apple shapes but probably not what's behind these distortions. Certain hormones have the purpose of directing where fat is placed on the body, and it is a distortion of this function that causes different body shapes.

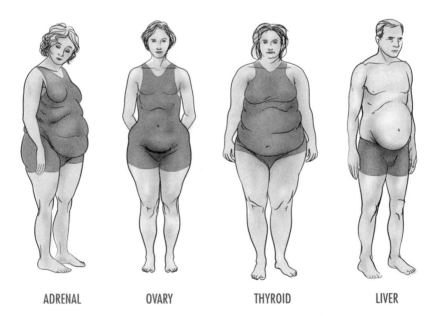

ADRENAL   OVARY   THYROID   LIVER

As mentioned earlier, the primary purpose of fat is not to be a cushion or insulation. It is a secondary reserve of energy, the primary one being sugar.

Fat means survival to the body because it is stored energy. The body has a tendency to hold fat around vital organs that are stressed as an act of protection against starvation. During pregnancy, the body will accumulate fat usually around the hips and thighs, as this will ensure extra fuel for the growing fetus.

I've been on a mission for many years to find the real underlying causes of health problems and stubborn weight, and I think you are going to like what I have found.

The distinctive quality of this program is the discovery that different body shapes are the result of specific correlating glandular problems (adrenals, ovaries, thyroid and liver). This program targets ALL of these problems, allowing for maximum weight loss. One can't just put everybody on the same foods and expect to be successful. Each person needs to eat and exercise for his or her specific gland weakness.

I have identified *four* different and distinctive types of weight problems.

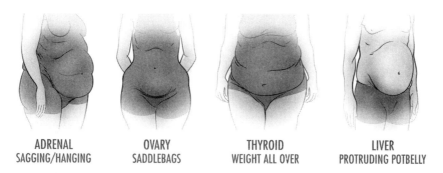

| ADRENAL | OVARY | THYROID | LIVER |
| SAGGING/HANGING | SADDLEBAGS | WEIGHT ALL OVER | PROTRUDING POTBELLY |

The outside of the body gives clues as to what's going on inside. In the case of the adrenal glands, the body when under stress will store energy (as fat) around the vital organs—in the abdomen. If there is an ovary problem, you'll see excess fat accumulate around the hips and thighs with a lower stomach bulge just under the bellybutton. When there is a weakness in the thyroid gland, because thyroid hormones are directed into all cells of the body, an overall appearance of weight gain will occur rather than in just one location. And when the liver is weak, fluid can leak into the sac around the abdomen, giving a "potbelly" appearance.

The Adrenal body shape is adipose tissue surrounding the organs in the abdomen (intra-abdominal fat) and is called a pendulous abdomen. The Latin derivation of *pendulous*, the verb *pendere*, means "to hang or sag." The Ovary body shape is more of an estrogen cellulite-type fat, which is superficial (just under the skin) and mostly below the bellybutton. People call this "saddlebags" with a lower stomach bulge. The Thyroid body shape is yet a different type of fat altogether. The weight is deposited all over the person's body and is not really fat but more of a waste-like substance that accumulates between the cells. This condition is known as myxedema, and it can be likened to a sponge that holds in liquid and will not release it. *Myx-* comes from the Greek word *myxa*, meaning "mucus" or "slime," and *edema* comes from the Greek *oidēma*, which means "swelling." Then there is the Liver body shape. This is not always a fat situation; it can be a fluid problem, where an accumulation of fluid is leaking into the abdomen.

You'll learn about these body types in detail in chapters 5 through 8.

Principle #2

Calories Are Insignificant Compared to Fat-Burning Hormones

You have probably been told that weight gain or obesity is caused by "consuming more calories than are burned" and the way to lose weight is to eat fewer calories. That is what I once believed too. But how do we explain the skinny guy who eats like a horse yet doesn't gain an ounce? And what about the overweight person who looks at food across the table and gains five pounds?

The real problem lies more in metabolism and the hormones that control it. When you cut calories, you can initially lose weight. But then it rebounds and you will gain back more later, especially in the stomach area, because "low calories" or "hunger" is the trigger for the fat-storing stress hormone. We'll get into that later.

Calories are units of energy in various foods.

Hormones look at food calories differently. Without having a good understanding of hormones, it might appear that *all* calories are the same and if you eat less you will of course weigh less. People who tell you this have not grasped the basic physiology of hormone interaction resulting from foods. And the obvious proof of this is that you probably have been cutting calories with minimal or no effect. A theory is only as true as it works.

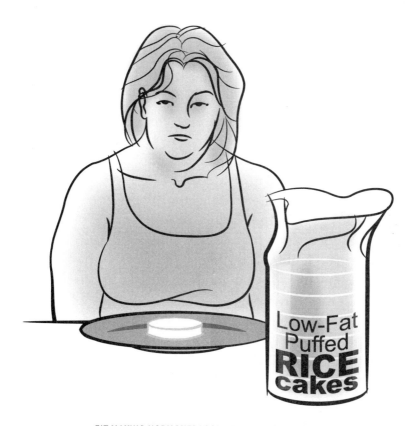

FAT-MAKING HORMONES LOOK AT CALORIES DIFFERENTLY

Even though fats have the densest calories, they are neutral when it comes to making fat. Sugar and refined carbohydrates, on the other hand, are huge triggers to fat-making hormones despite having fewer calories than fats. And although protein has calories, consuming the right amount of protein will trigger fat-burning hormones. The "right amount" is based on your body type, which I'll explain in chapter 11.

Principle #3

You Have to Be Healthy Before You Can Lose Weight

You have no doubt heard that you should lose weight so you can be healthier, because obesity is a health risk causing heart disease, diabetes, arthritis and stroke. Right? People have been pushing the idea that *fat* directly causes these other problems.

This is not true!

I found it is just the opposite. You need to be healthy first before you can actually lose weight. You are fat because some area of your body is unhealthy. In other words, heart disease, diabetes, arthritis, stroke AND obesity are all the result (symptoms) of the same thing—an unhealthy body. Somehow, someone has assigned *obesity* as a primary cause or a disease, when in reality it is an effect or result of something else.

The problem with making it a disease is now it gets treated with medication, and if some nonmedical practitioner treats it, he or she could be practicing medicine without a license.

If you have stubborn weight problems, you have unhealthy hormones. You can't be fat and healthy at the same time.

The body can't and won't release fat until it is at a certain level of health. It shouldn't surprise you to learn *why* your body is holding on so dearly to fat if you understand the purpose of fat. It is a survival mechanism, and the body will not let go of fat until the source of stress or the threat to survival is gone—in other words, until the body is healthy.

You could force your body to lose weight by taking an appetite suppressant, drinking canned diet shakes with high-fructose corn syrup or starving yourself, but this would not be the optimum solution, as it would give you a bigger problem down the road. Jumping in and fixing your weight problem with dieting (cutting calories) and typical exercise, without first finding out *what* problem you have, would not be the best approach either. Losing weight would be a lot more difficult because you'd be focusing on the wrong goal—weight loss. The correct goal is to create healthier glands and hormones. The weight loss will then occur as a benefit of having a healthier body.

So here is what I want you to change, right now. From now on, NO LONGER TREAT SYMPTOMS!

Your weight is a symptom, not the cause. Shift all your energy and attention to fixing the cause by creating a healthy body and the symptom of weight *will no longer be a problem.* Can you imagine an auto mechanic spending his entire time trying to cover up the clanking sound in the engine of your car? We've applied this principle to thousands of people and it works every single time.

This brings up the next question: Which foods have the capacity to create the greatest health for your body?

Let's first take the reverse of that: What condition is the most unhealthy? The answer, of course, is cancer. And are there foods that could potentially inhibit or reverse cancer? Yes sir! Anticancer foods would be the healthiest foods you could possibly eat to create health and burn fat. I include these foods in step one of the eating plan, beginning on page 145.

I think the entire concept of an unhealthy gland or hormone causing a distorted body has been given little attention for this one reason: Many doctors base their entire diagnosis on blood tests. These are fine for diagnosing major disease states but not for detecting subclinical gland and hormone imbalances. You have to have major liver damage before positive findings show up on blood tests. The same is true of the adrenal glands.[1] Your body tends to keep the blood chemistry constant no matter what.

"My Hormone Blood Tests Are Normal"

I can't tell you how many times I've heard, "My hormone blood tests came out normal but I have all the symptoms and I'm still fat." Let me explain something. Rarely are the relationships between the hormones looked at. For instance, if the adrenals overproduce their stress hormones, the important fat-burning hormone — growth hormone — can be suppressed. If your ovary has a cyst on it, excessive estrogen can

---

1. This and other numbered references throughout the chapters can be viewed in the reference section beginning on page 301.

be produced, which can block the thyroid and create thyroid symptoms (hair loss, overweight, brittle nails, etc.).

Eighty percent of thyroid hormone activation occurs through the liver, so a person with thyroid symptoms could have normal thyroid hormones but have liver damage; and failing to look deeper at the relationship between these two organs, the person's focus could be on the wrong problem and they could end up trying to resolve a secondary situation for years with no success.

So, if you have problems yet tests keep coming out normal, ask your doctor to evaluate more broadly. If you only check the thyroid hormones, you can miss the adrenal, ovary or even the pituitary hormones. Without really evaluating the hugely significant importance of hormone interactions, a person is stuck "treating the symptoms."

But please realize I am not an endocrinologist, and this book is not about diagnosing or treating any medical disease or condition. It is more an education to inform you how your body works, with emphasis on the fat-burning effects of hormones through food and exercise. I believe it is important to inform people how their own bodies work, since the word *doctor* means "teacher."

Excess fat is a symptom, simply the tip of the iceberg, not the actual cause. You could say the most important discovery has been that the majority of people are attempting to solve the wrong problem. Have you ever tried to solve the wrong thing? This leads to wasted time and energy with no results!

Let's take a look at the real problem — the failure of your fat cells to release energy. To solve this problem, you need to first know what a fat cell is and its purpose.

What Is Fat?

Though not commonly realized, fat is the largest endocrine gland in the body. Being an important part of body composition, adipose tissue (fat) accepts a lot of hormonal signals and is able, as well, to produce and secrete hormones and hormone-like substances.

Fat contains potential energy. *Potential* means "capable of being or becoming; possible but not actual." Fat is potential energy because it is fuel that has not yet become energy. It is stored energy or reserve energy.

The truth is you're not really *fat*; you just have too much potential energy. Sounds better, doesn't it? You should get a T-shirt that says, "I'm not FAT. I have lots of POTENTIAL ENERGY"!

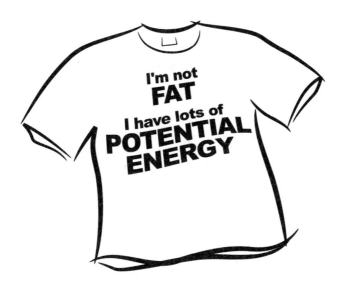

Fat is similar to money in the bank. You go to work every day and produce something for your paycheck. You then pay your bills; anything extra goes into your bank account. Hopefully you don't spend everything you make and you have some extra reserves in the bank. You have access to this money through an ATM card, credit card or your bank account number and proper identification. Fat is equivalent to the body's reserve bank account. I know what you are saying right now: "I must be a billionaire!"

But how could you have all this extra potential energy and at the same time be even the slightest bit tired? You might even crave energy—in the form of breads, pasta, cereals, chips or chocolate. It's a weird situation—having tons of stored potential energy, yet you can't release it. That is because this stored energy is *unavailable* to you. You need a specific key to release the fat and turn it into energy. Well, guess what? You already have the keys; they are your own hormones. To do this, though, you have to understand these keys and use the right ones. You have roughly 600 hormone keys. Of this number, six are fat burning and three are fat storing. If any of the three fat-storing hormones are active, they will nullify ALL six fat-burning hormones. The secret is to activate the six and keep the three inactive.

Principle #4

Environmental Hormones and Chemicals Mimic Your Hormones

If you want to know why your weight problem is becoming worse, you don't have to look far. You are presently being exposed to synthetic environmental hormones on a daily basis. The meats and meat products we eat come from animals that have been given hormones — chickens, turkeys, cattle and fish. Certain groups will tell you there is no proof that these man-made hormones administered to animals have any effect on our bodies. Yet if you go overseas to countries that don't use these hormones, people are thinner — Europeans especially.

Another interesting observation is that chemicals such as pesticides and insecticides have the ability to act like hormones in our bodies. Your food is heavily sprayed with these toxic chemicals.

The Environmental Protection Agency has a name for these chemicals; collectively they're called *endocrine disruptors*, meaning any chemicals that mimic, block or otherwise disrupt the normal function of hormones. You'll learn more about these in chapter 3.

> I talked to a Russian cab driver recently while being taken to the airport. I asked him, "Are people in Russia fat compared to Americans?" He said, "No, I've never seen so many fat people in my life since moving to America. In Russia, you only see someone fat with some sort of sickness." In Russia, he used to be a driver for a chicken factory, so I asked him if they use growth hormones to grow chickens as they do in America. He said no and replied that they just keep the lights on and provide lots of food for the chickens and they keep eating 24/7. He said, "You Americans have restaurants and food places open when you should be

sleeping—and Americans are like those chickens that can't stop eating." I then asked him about drinking vodka, because I was curious about damage to the liver. I wanted to know if Russian people have protruding bellies, and, sure enough, he said they do. The Liver body shape shows up as a potbelly.

Principle #5

You Have to Heal Your Glands and Hormones to KEEP the Weight Off

The aim of this book is to change your viewpoint of the primary goal from losing weight to complete healing of your weak gland — achieving stable weight loss. Let's focus on the real problem!

The key to keeping the weight off is achieving full rejuvenation of your glands and hormones — in other words, doing the program long enough for your body to fully heal. Not completely fixing the true problem (unstable glands) causes the problem to come right back.

When certain glands get sick, the hormones they produce can physically dissolve the muscles in your legs, buttocks and arms, leaving you with shrunken, weak and flaccid muscles. These destructive hormones literally eat up muscle proteins, turning them into fat around your midsection. So, instead of using fat reserves for fuel, your body uses muscle proteins, which are turned into sugar as fuel, leaving you fat, flabby, stressed and weak.

As a person starts the program and these glands heal, the muscles need to be rebuilt. These muscles are a bit heavier than fat; therefore the person's weight might not initially change, even though their clothes feel looser. Before the body will burn fat, it has to build back this lost muscle tissue.

I had a female patient who was over 350 pounds. In the first month she didn't lose any weight at all, yet her energy, sleeping, digestion and muscle strength were greatly improved. Most people would be discouraged by this, since they'd be looking at the weight indicator only. In my mind she was right on track, because the second month she lost 23 pounds, and by the third month she had lost a total of 61 pounds. Her body had to grow protein in her leg muscles before burning fat, and protein weighs more than fat.

I have found that fat will come off in direct relation to the health of your hormones. Because fat, to the body, is survival (reserve energy), the body will not release this energy until it is sure it's in safe mode. As can be seen in the diagram below, while healing is occurring it might take some time before your body is healthy enough to burn fat and lose weight. It could take about a month before the weight starts to come off. However, your energy will be up, you'll feel stronger, have fewer cravings, and your overall mood will improve.

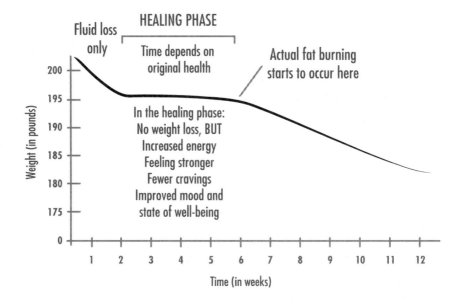

Adipose tissue is *only* used when absolutely necessary — after the sugar fuel has been exhausted. The body *always* uses stored sugar or dietary sugar as a priority before tapping into fat fuel. This is the principal reason why people are not losing weight. Most of them are running their bodies on sugar fuel. You must deplete your sugar reserves BEFORE you can tap into your fat reserves.

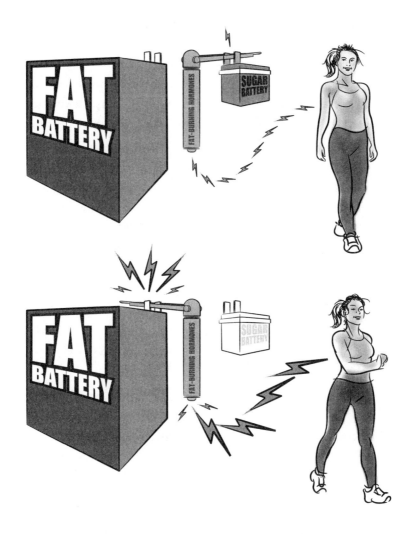

How Do You Know It's Working?

The best way to know if your organs and glands are healing and the program is working is not just by weight loss but by other positive health indicators—improved energy, better quality of sleep, better digestion, clothes fitting more loosely, more muscle strength, better nail and hair quality, decreased cravings, and overall feelings of well-being. These indicators give you the valuable feedback that your body is healing.

In other words, you need to shift your goal from "losing weight" to "attaining health," since only through this can you fully reach your ideal weight, as overweight is a symptom of an unhealthy body.

It's amazing what obese people are fed in certain obesity clinics—powdered sweet chocolate mixtures with very low calories, diet pills, appetite suppressants and B₁₂ shots. They will experience a very temporary weight reduction, but these treatments will bring a person's health downward in the long run.

> A woman came to my clinic with constant burping after consuming one of these powdered mixtures. Burping means gallbladder and liver problems. It's one thing to not have a successful weight loss program, but it's another thing to worsen the entire situation.

Principle #6

Fat-Burning and Fat-Storing Hormones Have Their Own Triggers

Hormones control metabolism and each one associated with fat burning and fat storing has its own triggers. Hormones are triggered or blocked by foods, exercise and other activities.

There are two things that can happen with these triggers. You can eat and exercise to stimulate fat burning or you can eat and exercise for fat storing. The huge hidden problem I discovered was that most people are nullifying the fat-burning hormones by using the wrong triggers. For instance, correct exercise might work if you can get seven hours of quality sleep per night, whereas poor or inadequate sleep will prevent fat burning. And just a little bit of sweet carbohydrate can set your fat burning back for a day. This is why "everything in moderation" doesn't work with fat burning. Another example is drinking wine at night, as alcohol is a gland (liver) destroyer and can set back fat burning for hours or days.

The more of these hormone triggers you implement correctly, the faster and easier weight loss will be. Therefore, instead of wasting time counting calories, use the hormone triggers.

You will learn all of these important triggers in detail in chapter 9.

Principle #7

Incorrect Exercise Prevents Fat Burning

Another key discovery has been that different body types need different kinds of exercise.

I'm sure you have heard the theory "You're fat because you just don't exercise enough." Well, if you have an Adrenal body type and you do hard-core exercise, you not only will prevent fat burning, your body might even get bigger. I see these people at the gym with their personal trainers working to lose weight for years with very little change. Exercise only works if your body has good adrenals. If you have an Adrenal body type, adding more exercise to an already stressed-out body is self-defeating. Adrenal types need very light, slow exercise.

On the other hand, if you have a Liver body type, the fat-burning hormones need to be stimulated intensely for weight loss to occur. If the exercise is too light or too slow, you get no effects. Exercising for your specific body type can be a big advantage in maximizing weight loss.

Many people have the idea that their fat is excess calories and all they need to do is burn these off through exercising. However, it's not the calories burned during exercise that are significant. It's the delayed fat-burning peaks that occur between 14 and 48 hours later[2]—but only if specific conditions are correct in regard to sleep and stress levels.

The Exercise Longer to Lose Weight Myth

This philosophy is currently being pushed heavily in gyms. I have had quite a few patients come to my office who were exercise enthusiasts. One woman not only was exercising two hours per day seven days per week but she also ran a 26-mile marathon — with *zero* weight loss. Talk about depressing!

Since the adrenals are the stress glands, if you have an Adrenal body shape, then the longer and harder you exercise, the less you will lose because you are triggering those darn stress hormones again — causing more belly fat.

So, there is a specific way you should be exercising to trigger fat burning, depending on your specific gland weakness.

In chapter 14, you will learn exactly how to use exercise for your body type.

Sticking to a Diet

This entire book could be summarized as teaching you how to get into and stay in healthy fat burning.

One of the greatest challenges for most individuals is sticking to a diet program once started. There is a very important reason for this. If you were to lose only two pounds a week from a diet, you might become discouraged and discontinue, especially if your friend down the street lost eight pounds per week. Fat loss unfortunately does not occur as quickly as fluid loss. But, on a positive note, many people have lots of water weight to lose, and losing that alone can hugely change the way someone looks. It might even be possible to lose six pounds of water weight per week for several weeks, but as soon as your water weight becomes normal, the weight loss for a person with a healthy metabolism is one to two pounds per week. If you don't know this, you can easily give up.

3

Hormones and
Your Body Shape

The hormonal system as a whole is called the endocrine system. If you look up the word *endocrine*, you will find it comes from *endo-*, a combining form that means "within" or "inner," and the Greek word *krinein*, which means "to separate." *Webster's New World Dictionary* then says, "see CRISIS." When you go to the word *crisis*, you find it comes from the same derivation, "to separate, discern." This is interesting because the endocrine system IS the system that discerns or determines threats to normal survival, keeping the body out of crisis via hormones.

If its survival is threatened in any way, the body will start to hold energy—which is the accumulation of fat. This is the body's attempt to keep you alive and surviving; and as long as the threat to survival remains, fat will be held on to tightly and will overdevelop to compensate for the lack of survival.

Many people think that the shape of a body is purely genetic and there is nothing that can be done about it. It is true that there are genetic tendencies. It is also true that hormonal imbalances will cause excessive distortions of accumulated fat in different locations around the body. An imbalance on the inside can show up on the outside.

Hormones do diminish as you age, but that is not the sole reason for your weight problem. Take a look around—younger people are getting fat too. Some of the fat-burning hormones are also the antiaging hormones. So the goal of this program is twofold: to help you lose weight and to make you younger.

The hormone system is very sensitive to environmental chemicals, especially growth hormones in the foods we eat. Our foods are injected with hormones; they are also sprayed with pesticides, which have the ability to mimic hormones. You have been swimming in a sea of toxic chemicals. Welcome to planet Earth!

When these chemicals enter the body, they plug up or interfere with hormone receptors. Glands make and send hormones. Cells then receive these in a similar way to a catcher in a baseball game. If you are born with 20,000 hormone receptors per cell and are constantly exposed to environmental growth hormone mimickers—chemicals such as pesticides and insecticides—eventually these block the receptors, leaving very few for hormone reception. It's like driving into New York City and trying to find a parking place. As you age, the chemical exposure accumulates until your system gets overwhelmed and can't burn fat anymore. But it's not just older people; young people get fat too due to this environmental toxicity factor.

What Is a Hormone?

A hormone can be defined simply as a chemical message produced by a gland in the body and sent through the bloodstream to another area where it causes some effect. For example, exercising can create fat-burning effects that last for 48 hours after the workout. There are over 600 different hormones in the body, each with a unique function. Fat burning, fat storing, appetite, sleep, hair and fingernail growth, fluid levels and joint repair are just a few examples of direct effects that hormones have on the body.

Hormones are the language of the body. Instead of words, hormones tell the body what to do, causing millions of effects each day. Glands create these messages; they both send and receive communications. Daily functions of the body are controlled mainly by hormones; for instance, they tell the heart how fast to pump and the bones how quickly to grow. If hormones become dysfunctional, a person could have osteoporosis (thinning of the bones) despite the amount of calcium consumed.

Each gland has its own purpose in regulating certain areas of the body. The adrenals, for instance, help the body to handle stress in all its different aspects. Imagine for a moment a person starting to slip on some water while stepping down a flight of stairs. The adrenal glands would send off adrenaline (stress response hormone), which would put the body in high gear and prepare it for intense stressful action. Or imagine if you accidentally stepped on a large rattlesnake in your backyard. Your adrenal hormone adrenaline would spike, increasing the heart rate, creating sensations of fear, and pumping out instant energy to ready the body to hightail it out of there!

Gland-Hormone Connection

There is always a two-way connection back and forth within a properly working hormonal system. Not only do the glands talk but the cells of the body's tissues need to be listening as well. Once a message is sent and received, the cells are supposed to send a message back to let the gland know that the request has been received and complied with.

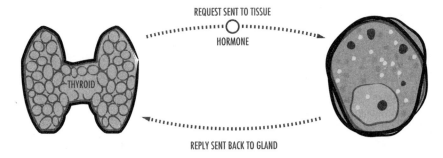

The word *communication* is derived from *common*, which means "shared equally." In order to have good communication you need an equal balance (50-50) of talking and listening. Hormone messages need to be received before they can work. If the receptors (mini-ears) within the body are blocked, there is no connection—similar to attempting to communicate to someone with earplugs.

The gland is giving the command or order "BURN FAT," and the fat cells are saying, "I'm sorry, did you say something?" And if the fat cells are not listening or are not receiving messages from the gland, no fat burning occurs.

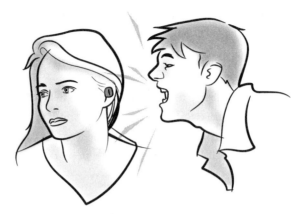

Or what about the person who talks so much that you tune them out? If because of a lack of response the gland starts "talking" too much, the fat cells eventually begin ignoring the fat-burning hormone messages.

Each gland, when in trouble, will create very specific bodily symptoms—the most noticeable one being a reshaping of the body. It takes years in some cases for hormone blood tests to show up as abnormal; and since all six fat-burning hormones have to do their job through the liver, there could be a normal level of hormones in the blood, yet the liver might not be activating them.

No matter how much you starve yourself, no matter how hard you exercise, if the fat-burning hormones are not being triggered, there will be no weight loss.

What Causes Gland and Liver Problems?

I've made some interesting observations with regard to why Americans are overweight. In northern Virginia where I practice, I have a melting pot of patients from all over the world. Upon surveying them, I have almost always found that they started becoming overweight when they moved to America. Some have told me that they lost weight when they went back home despite calorie intake or fat in their diets. This led me to evaluate the differences and similarities between America and other countries. Yes, people in other countries consume less fast foods and eat more fresh and natural foods, but they don't seem to be eating less fatty foods or lower calorie foods. They might also be getting more exercise; but then again, despite getting plenty of exercise, many Americans are not able to lose weight. So we can't just blame it all on "You're eating too much," or "You're not exercising," or "You're getting old."

What is the big difference or the real common denominator?

There is one significant factor I'd like to discuss. In America we fatten cattle, chickens and other animals via hormones. We give them estrogen and growth hormone to make them fatter. Even farm-raised fish are fed hormones. Well, if you consume turkey meat from turkeys that have been given hormones from birth, is it possible that some of the residue from the hormones could leach out in your body? If hormones can cause turkeys to look butterball size, is it possible that your body could also become butterball size?

Due to the presence of hormones in our food supply, we are seeing girls develop larger breasts and start their menstrual cycles at an increasingly younger age. Young boys are even developing extra breast tissue. This alone tells us that estrogen levels must be higher. Young girls with excessive sex drives may also have been exposed to estrogens in their diets.[1] Growth hormone, used in animal foods such as commercial milk, seems to be having an effect on our children as well—bigger feet especially. And I have observed women gaining weight when they go on the birth control pill or on hormone replacement therapy—again more estrogen.

Estrogen makes the fat layer around a female body. Fat cells also produce estrogen. Estrogen can inhibit thyroid and liver function.

Don't worry—it gets worse!

The Environmental Protection Agency (EPA) is doing major research on the effects of toxins called *endocrine disruptors* in both humans and wildlife.[2]

An endocrine disruptor is an environmental poison that mimics, blocks or otherwise disrupts the normal function of hormones.[3]

Examples of endocrine disruptors are
- pesticides: pest killers
- insecticides: insect killers
- herbicides: weed killers
- fungicides: fungus killers
- plastics
- solvents
- heavy metals

(The suffix -*cide* comes from the Latin word *caedere*, which means "to kill.")

The EPA has found that 90–95 percent of all pesticide residues are found in meat and dairy products.[4]

These chemicals act as if they were hormones. They have the ability to interfere with the binding of hormones. If hormones are keys and cell receptors the keyholes, endocrine disruptors can fit into these holes and block our hormones from functioning. Over time as a person ages and accumulates exposure to these chemicals, the receptors that are supposed to receive hormones get plugged, reducing hormone communication. This explains why hormones can lose their effectiveness and become resistant or stubborn. In other words, the key (hormone) can't fit into the keyhole (receptor) anymore.

METHODS OF HORMONE MISCOMMUNICATION

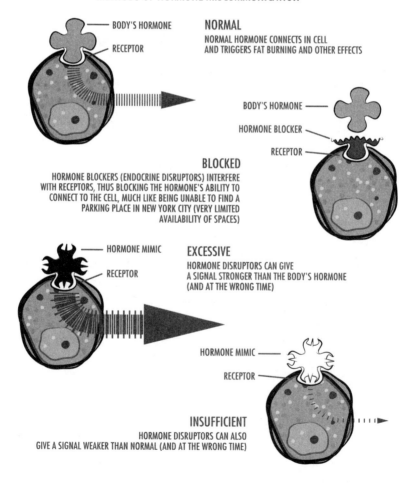

BODY'S HORMONE

RECEPTOR

NORMAL
NORMAL HORMONE CONNECTS IN CELL
AND TRIGGERS FAT BURNING AND OTHER EFFECTS

BODY'S HORMONE

HORMONE BLOCKER

RECEPTOR

BLOCKED
HORMONE BLOCKERS (ENDOCRINE DISRUPTORS) INTERFERE
WITH RECEPTORS, THUS BLOCKING THE HORMONE'S ABILITY TO
CONNECT TO THE CELL, MUCH LIKE BEING UNABLE TO FIND A
PARKING PLACE IN NEW YORK CITY (VERY LIMITED
AVAILABILITY OF SPACES)

HORMONE MIMIC

RECEPTOR

EXCESSIVE
HORMONE DISRUPTORS CAN GIVE
A SIGNAL STRONGER THAN THE BODY'S HORMONE
(AND AT THE WRONG TIME)

HORMONE MIMIC

RECEPTOR

INSUFFICIENT
HORMONE DISRUPTORS CAN ALSO
GIVE A SIGNAL WEAKER THAN NORMAL (AND AT THE WRONG TIME)

Another point regarding endocrine disruptors is that even tiny amounts can create hormone damage. It doesn't take much.

Schools, restaurants, golf courses, yards, foods, etc., are sprayed with chemicals that mimic estrogen. These toxins usually accumulate in only one or two organs.[5]

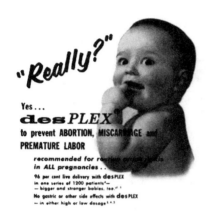

Between 1938 and 1970, doctors prescribed an artificial estrogen named diethylstilbestrol, or DES, to prevent miscarriages in millions of pregnant women. It was not until 30 years later that doctors discovered that DES had caused miscarriages, a rare form of cervical cancer, and many other health-related problems. One round of DES was equivalent to over 5,000 birth control pills. This was also the main growth hormone being given to animals during the same time.

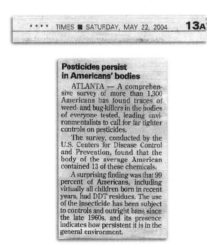

DDT, another chemical that mimics hormones, was found in recent years to be stored in the fat tissues of over 99 percent of children (May 22, 2004) despite being banned in 1969. Where is this coming from? We are allowed to sell it to third-world countries such as Mexico and Chile. Take a wild guess where we purchase our fruits and vegetables in the winter months.

These endocrine disruptors are also carcinogens. If you read any textbook on toxicology (study of poisons), you'll find these terms are synonymous. Carcinogens are those substances capable of causing cancer.

The word *cancer* has an interesting history. The cancer first found by the Greek physician Hippocrates was breast cancer, and the blood vessels that spread around the breast looked like crab legs; hence the Greek derivation *karkinos*, meaning "crab."

The reason you probably haven't heard much of this information broadly promoted is because it's difficult to prove. Carcinogens usually have a latency period of 30 or more years after initial exposure before tumors or cancer is observed. This is why it took 30 years to show up in daughters of mothers who took DES. These chemicals accumulate insidiously in certain tissues over the years, and since they compete with your hormones, the hormonal effects become less and less and the hormones can't quite connect to do their function.

Antifat-Making-Hormone Foods

The food plan I will be explaining later in the book has as one of its goals reducing in your food supply chemicals that mimic estrogen (fat-making hormone). Certain foods increase estrogen and others decrease it. There's one group of foods that is antiestrogen and antitoxin, called cruciferous (cabbage, broccoli, cauliflower, radish, kale, Brussels sprouts, etc.). *Cruciferous* comes from the Latin word *crux*, meaning "cross," since the flowers of these vegetables are shaped like a cross. If we're dealing with chemicals in the body, it makes sense to consume as many of these vegetables as possible or take them in whole-food supplement form.

To make a natural cleaning fluid for washing vegetables, mix one-third of a cup of apple cider vinegar in a gallon of water. This will remove some superficial chemicals, although nothing can remove the internal chemicals. Also, break off and discard the outer leaves of leafy vegetables.

Trim the fat from meat and the skin from poultry and fish if they are commercial. Also, if given a choice between commercial fish and commercial meat, go for the fish. It takes 60 pounds of pesticide-sprayed feed and hay to produce 1 pound of edible beef, not to mention growth hormones given throughout the lifetime of the cattle. It takes only 1 pound of feed to produce 1 pound of edible fish — hence fewer hormone-disrupting chemicals.

Coffee

Drinking two cups of coffee each day means buying some 18 pounds of beans each year — the total annual yield of 12 coffee trees. To keep those trees productive, coffee farmers apply 12 pounds of fertilizers and pesticides every year. Even though this program is going to recommend not drinking coffee, during the transition period I recommend consuming organic coffee. Coffee also contains caffeine and is damaging to your adrenal glands, a factor that can keep you from burning fat.

Organic means without the use of chemical fertilizers, pesticides, fungicides, herbicides and insecticides. When you read labels, you want to make sure they say *organic*, not *natural*. These are not the same.

Natural, in legal terminology, only means that those foods are not treated with chemicals during processing. *Natural* can mean many different things but it doesn't mean without pesticides or insecticides. I'm not saying you have to start eating 100 percent organic foods tomorrow. However, I would recommend eating at least 50 percent organic foods.

Now, you are not going to go to your friend's house for dinner and say, "You know, um . . . I recently read Dr. Berg's book and um . . . I noticed that that meal you're about to serve me is filled with pesticides, insecticides, herbicides, heavy metals, antibiotics and growth hormones. . . . And that tuna has mercury in it. . . . I hope you don't mind — I brought my own food in this bag here." You wouldn't do that; it's not socially accepted — you'd never be invited over again. Maybe that's why no one invites me to dinner anymore.

Fat-Burning and Fat-Storing Hormones

In order to understand the fat-burning hormones that trigger weight loss, you might want to know what these are. The following list gives not only the fat-burning hormones but also the fat-storing hormones, which you want to avoid triggering.

Fat-Burning Hormones

Growth Hormone (GH)

Growth hormone is made by a gland in your brain called the pituitary. Once made, it travels down to and works through the liver. This is a fat-burning, lean-muscle-building hormone. One of its key functions is building up cartilage and collagen. Without growth hormone, your joints and muscles fall apart and you age more quickly, as it's also an antiaging hormone. GH regulates fuel between meals and is active as well during the the night while you sleep. Poor liver function affects GH function. It is stimulated by protein and intense exercise. Interestingly, it is *not* triggered by light exercise.

Insulin-like Growth Factor (IGF)

IGF is made by the liver and is triggered by growth hormone. Its basic function is giving the body fuel between meals and it does this through releasing stored sugar and fat; thus it is a fat-burning hormone. Insulin is the opposing hormone to control body fuel while you are eating. IGF is stimulated when the stomach is empty, which is why Liver body types should not be eating or snacking between meals. When the liver is damaged, this hormone decreases, putting added stress on the pancreas to supply fuel through raised insulin.

Glucagon

Glucagon raises blood sugar by tapping into the fat reserves and is therefore called a fat-burning hormone. It has an opposing action to insulin. It helps control blood sugar between meals and is stimulated by dietary protein and intense exercise. However, if excess protein is eaten, insulin will be elevated and will blunt this hormone.

Adrenaline

Adrenaline is the main hormone that releases fat from the fat cells. It has many additional functions to prepare the body for stressful situations: mental alertness, increased heart rate, metabolic rate, blood pressure, etc. It is triggered by exercise.

Thyroid Hormones (T3 and T4)

These hormones control the speed of your metabolism. They trigger metabolism by increasing the size and number of the cellular energy factories, called mitochondria. The faster the metabolism, the thinner the person is. People with insufficient thyroid hormone secretion are overweight. One way to inhibit these hormones is to cut calories or skip meals.

Testosterone

Testosterone is made by the adrenal glands, the testicles, and even the ovaries. This fat-burning hormone assists in giving you lean muscles and is involved in sex drive and male characteristics. If a female has high testosterone, she gets facial hair, a deeper voice and male-pattern baldness. It is stimulated by exercise and countered by estrogen.

Fat-Storing Hormones

Insulin

Insulin is made by the pancreas; its function is to lower blood sugar after meals. It will cause the cells to absorb sugar as fuel and will convert the rest to fat and cholesterol. Insulin works with IGF and glucagon to keep fuel constant in the blood; so when IGF and glucagon go down, insulin must go up and vice versa. In the presence of insulin, you will not be able to burn fat. Sugar triggers insulin.

Estrogen

(From the Greek word *oistros*, meaning "mad desire," + *genēs*, "born")

Estrogen is responsible for the female characteristics, menstrual cycle and changes of the uterus and breasts. It provides the fat layer around a female body, especially around the outer thighs. The reason women tend to have more fat than men lies in the fact that women have over a thousand times the concentration of estrogen receptors that men have.

Cortisol

This is an important hormone produced by the adrenal glands, which is activated by stress of all kinds. It is anti-inflammatory and releases sugar from the liver and muscles into the blood as an instant fuel source for stressful events. Cortisol is classified as a fat burner; however, it also has an indirect fat-storing effect when it turns body-muscle proteins into sugar fuel, since this forces insulin to deal with the excess sugar in the bloodstream, producing weight gain in the midsection.

Fat-Burning-Tracker Coach

One of the very successful tools we use in our clinic is an Internet program called the Fat-Burning-Tracker Coach, and this benefit is now available to you as a companion to this book at http://www.fbtcoach.com/. Through this program, you can have a trained person (health coach) giving you personal supervision and closely analyzing your diet. You will also get reports and graphs of your hormone responses to food, showing whether you are in fat burning or not.*

An example of one of the graphs provided by this program is displayed on the next page. Twenty-four hours a day your body is in one of four conditions or states. It can be in *fat-burning mode,* which is the optimum level seen at the top of the graph, or in *fat-storing mode*—the worst condition—shown at the bottom of the graph. You can also be at levels in between.

---

* For additional information, see the resources section, page 313, and Fat-Burning Tracker Web Support, page 331.

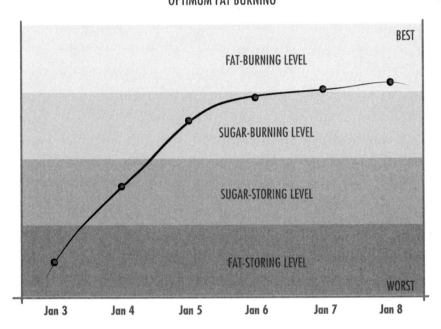

The Fat-Burning Tracker extracts all the foods you eat every day and associates the hormone interactions with these, so that you can get a bird's-eye view of where you are at and what you need to work on.

4

Finding Your Body Type

Take the Quiz to Find Out Which Body Type You Are!

Each body type has its own characteristics. Taking this quiz helps to zero in on your specific type. You might find, as you do the quiz, that you answer yes to questions in more than one body type and so think, "I'm mixed between a few types." This could be true, but there is always a primary; most people have a primary type that is causing secondary symptoms. One type can create problems for another type, as you will learn in the last section of this chapter. When one hormone increases, others can decrease. The purpose of this quiz is not to diagnose you. The purpose is to inform you about your body and help to find possible areas of weakness based on how glands behave when they are stressed.

The Body Type Quiz

Before you do the complete quiz, there are several questions upfront that will quickly find out if the liver and gallbladder are involved. If the answers to these questions are yes, then you might be on the Liver Enhancement for a longer period of time.

If you answer YES to ANY of the seven points below, you need foods that support the liver and thyroid. You do not need to go through the quiz — you already have your answer.

	YES	NO
1. Have had your gallbladder removed	❏	❏
2. History of gallstones	❏	❏
3. Can't lose weight on high-protein diets (e.g., Atkins)	❏	❏
4. Dislike consuming lots of heavy protein-type foods	❏	❏
5. Inability to digest fatty or greasy foods, especially at night	❏	❏
6. History of liver problems	❏	❏
7. Protruding, distended belly—potbelly	❏	❏

DIRECTIONS: Circle one letter (A, B, C or D) in each question below. If there is more than one symptom that you are experiencing within a question, circle the one that is most prominent.

For women who are menopausal or post-menopausal, the Ovary (D) questions should be answered from the viewpoint of having had, or not had, previous problems with or a history of the condition mentioned.

1. Do you . . .	A. crave sweets, breads and pasta?	a. Thyroid
	B. crave salt (pretzels, cheese puffs or salty peanuts) or chocolate?	b. Adrenal
	C. crave deep-fried foods or potato chips?	c. Liver
	D. crave ice cream, cream cheese, sour cream or milk?	d. Ovary
2. Are you . . .	A. often depressed or feeling hopeless?	a. Thyroid
	B. a worrier or often anxious and nervous?	b. Adrenal
	C. irritable, moody, grouchy, in the morning?	c. Liver
	D. moody/irritable at certain times of the month?	d. Ovary
3. Do you . . .	A. feel better on fruits and berries?	a. Thyroid
	B. need coffee or stimulants to wake up?	b. Adrenal
	C. experience a tight feeling over your right lower stomach area or rib cage?	c. Liver
	D. experience constipation during menstruation?	d. Ovary

4. Do you have . . .	A. brittle nails with vertical ridges?	a. Thyroid
	B. facial hair as a female?	b. Adrenal
	C. pain/tightness in right shoulder area?	c. Liver
	D. pain in right or left lower back/hip area?	d. Ovary
5. Do you have . . .	A. a weight problem more evenly distributed?	a. Thyroid
	B. a pendulous abdomen, meaning hanging, sagging and loose?	b. Adrenal
	C. a protruding abdomen (potbelly)?	c. Liver
	D. excess fat on thighs and hips (saddlebags) and a lower stomach bulge?	d. Ovary
6. Do you have . . .	A. dry skin, especially hands and around elbows?	a. Thyroid
	B. swollen ankles—socks leave creases on ankles?	b. Adrenal
	C. flaky skin or dandruff in eyebrows and scalp?	c. Liver
	D. menstrual cyclic hair loss?	d. Ovary
7. Do you have . . .	A. indentations on both sides of your tongue where the tongue meets the teeth?	a. Thyroid
	B. atrophy (shrinkage) of the thigh muscles with difficulty getting up from a seated position?	b. Adrenal
	C. dark yellow urine?	c. Liver
	D. hot flashes?	d. Ovary
8. Do you have . . .	A. a loss of hair on the outer third of the eyebrows?	a. Thyroid
	B. dizziness when getting up too quickly?	b. Adrenal
	C. hot or swollen feet?	c. Liver
	D. menstrual cyclic brain fog?	d. Ovary

9. Do you have . . .	A. to sleep with socks on at night because of feeling cold?	a. Thyroid
	B. chronic inflammation in body?	b. Adrenal
	C. headaches or head feels heavy in morning?	c. Liver
	D. excessive menstrual bleeding?	d. Ovary
10. Do you have . . .	A. puffiness around eyes?	a. Thyroid
	B. an unusual feeling of being "out of breath" while climbing stairs?	b. Adrenal
	C. skin problems (psoriasis, eczema, brown spots)?	c. Liver
	D. low sex drive?	d. Ovary
11. Do you have . . .	A. excessive skin sagging under arms?	a. Thyroid
	B. twitching under or on top of left eyelid?	b. Adrenal
Are you . . .	C. not a morning person, yet feel more awake at night?	c. Liver
Do you have . . .	D. weight gain one week before menstrual period?	d. Ovary
12. Do you . . .	A. have dry hair and hair loss?	a. Thyroid
	B. wake up in the middle of the night (2:00–3:00 a.m.)?	b. Adrenal
	C. have a deep crevice (deep crease appearance) down center of tongue and/or a white film on tongue?	c. Liver
	D. have an upper body which is thinner than your lower body?	d. Ovary
13. Do you experience . . .	A. not being able to maintain curls in your hair after using a curling iron?	a. Thyroid
	B. cramps in the calves at night?	b. Adrenal
	C. more itching at night?	c. Liver
	D. water retention at certain times of the month?	d. Ovary

14. Do you . . .	A. become excessively tired in the early evening (7:30–8:00 p.m.) and more awake in the early morning?	a. Thyroid
	B. have a more active bladder at night than during the day?	b. Adrenal
	C. have a yellow tint in the whites of your eyes?	c. Liver
	D. have a history of ovarian or breast cysts?	d. Ovary
15. Do you have . . .	A. a lack of get-up-and-go (vitality)?	a. Thyroid
	B. calcium issues or deposits—bursitis, tendonitis, kidney stones, heal spurs, early cataracts?	b. Adrenal
	C. major moodiness if you skip a meal?	c. Liver
	D. difficulty losing weight after pregnancy?	d. Ovary
16. Do you have . . .	A. a history of being on low-calorie diets?	a. Thyroid
	B. low tolerance for stressful situations, get easily irritable and on edge?	b. Adrenal
	C. stiffness and pain more in the right shoulder and right side of neck?	c. Liver
	D. pain and tightness in one knee, worse during menstrual cycle?	d. Ovary

Count up the total of each:

Total A. Thyroid _____   Total B. Adrenal _____

Total C. Liver +_____   Total D. Ovary + _____

= _____   = _____

Liver & Thyroid Eating & Exercise Plan   Adrenal & Ovary Eating & Exercise Plan

There are two basic eating and exercise plans, as seen on the previous page. However, everyone will first start with the Liver Enhancement. Based on these results, you will then go to either the Liver & Thyroid plan or the Adrenal & Ovary plan.

Your next step is to start reading about your specific body type (the one you answered yes to the most) and then read the chapters on the other types that might apply. You could find you are a combination of two or more body types. But everyone has a primary body type; the others are just secondary.

If you were not able to clearly determine your body type from the quiz, look through the symptoms listed for each body type at the end of chapters 5, 6, 7 and 8 to see which symptoms you have the most of— Adrenal, Ovary, Thyroid or Liver.

The best way to be really certain of your type is through the eating plan. If you do very well on the Liver Enhancement in chapter 10, you'll be more of a Liver or Thyroid; and if you do better with additional protein, then you'll know you are more of an Adrenal or Ovary.

Why Am I a Mixed Type?

As mentioned earlier in the chapter, most people have a primary problem and many secondary issues. For instance, an overactive ovary can inhibit the thyroid, creating weakness and symptoms in the thyroid, yet the real problem is in the ovary. If the liver is blocked, the thyroid is automatically inhibited because 80 percent of thyroid function occurs through the liver. If the adrenal glands are overworking and producing excess hormones, growth hormone from the liver will be inhibited, which will force the pancreas to produce more insulin, causing increased fat in the abdomen. So you can see the complexity of these relationships and the importance of finding the root cause.

5
The Adrenal Type

The Adrenal Glands

You have two adrenal glands, one located on top of each kidney.

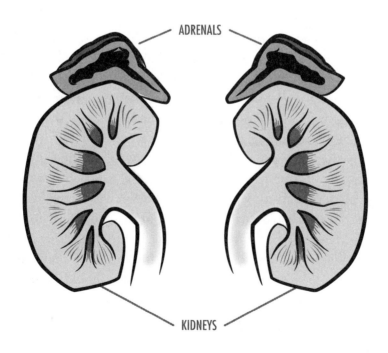

THE ADRENAL GLANDS

One of the main functions of these glands is countering stress by the production of several hormones. The adrenals don't know the difference between physical and mental stress; they treat both with the same stress hormones. Every type of stress influences these glands[1]—injury, infection, divorce, financial stress, job-related stress, irritable people, drugs and medication, surgery, pain, illness, poison ivy, extreme cold or heat, giving birth, menstrual cycle, staring into computer monitors, eating junk foods, starvation diets, and babysitting 15 small children under the age of five for over 13 hours.

The adrenals have many other functions, from anti-inflammatory actions (ridding the body of pain and swelling) and immune system protection to balancing fluid and salt levels, and controlling minerals (such as potassium), rapid heart rate and sleep and awake cycles. They even act as backup organs for the ovaries during menopause.

The following is a description of what happens when the adrenal glands do not function properly.

The Adrenal type I am about to describe is the result of excessive adrenal hormone production. I will cover adrenal hormone deficiency as well.

Excess fat in both the midsection (buffalo-like torso) and the face can occur from overreaction of this gland. In the midsection, the fat forms primarily in and around the abdominal organs and sags downward over the belly. Another term for this stomach is *pendulous*, meaning "hanging loosely," "sagging." This is different from the Liver body shape, which is a potbelly or a protruding stomach like a water balloon, while in the Ovary body shape the person has a small bulge below the bellybutton.

The majority of Americans hold weight in the stomach area more than any other place (which could come from the adrenals or the liver). There are different degrees of adrenal problems, but many of them do not show up on blood tests until they are well advanced into dangerous stages. The adrenal glands are set on a timing mechanism in the brain; therefore testing the blood or saliva for adrenal hormones should be done every 4 hours through a 24-hour period (cortisol test).

The Adrenal Type

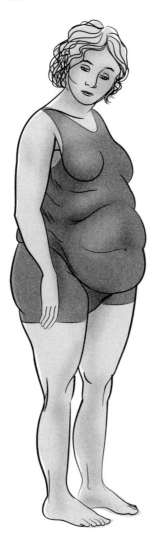

SAGGING, HANGING MIDSECTION WEIGHT WITH THIN ARMS AND LEGS

A fat pad can develop in the lower neck and upper back area, called a "buffalo hump."[2] I believe the reason the body creates this is to anchor the belly so you don't fall forward.

Fat accumulation in the face gives a round or "moon face" appearance.[3] The face also has redness because of weakened blood vessels.

Reddish purple striations (strips or bands resembling stretch marks) can appear on the stomach, thighs, buttocks, arms and breasts as well.

This type of individual generally has a large midsection with thin arms and legs. The reason is very interesting. The adrenal stress hormone cortisol breaks down leg muscle and turns it into sugar. This is a stress response by the body to supply quick energy; if you were being chased by a lion, you would need this energy. This sugar, if not completely burned up, will be converted to fat around the belly where the vital organs lie. The person's legs could eventually become thinner and weaker too, particularly at the knees. Cortisol will also take muscle from the buttocks, causing loss of tone in that area.

A common problem with the Adrenal type is the inability to fit into clothing, especially around the waist. Some people even wear elastic bands to hold the belly in, but this can constrict vital organs within the abdomen.

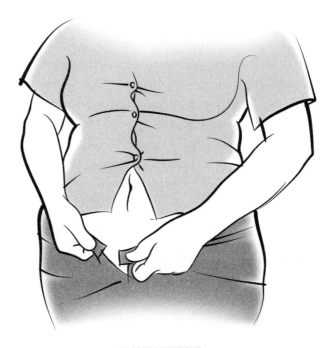

MIDSECTION WEIGHT

The pictures below show the changes from a normal body shape through the progressive stages of the Adrenal type.

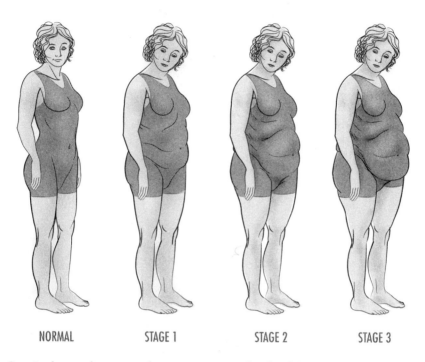

NORMAL   STAGE 1   STAGE 2   STAGE 3

Cortisol can be very destructive on the body's proteins, especially bone tissue, leading to "thinning of the bones" (osteoporosis). It steals these proteins to use them as fuel, and during stress mode the body will go after any type of fuel, even your own body tissue. This might explain why some people have difficulty losing weight on high-protein diets. High protein is supposed to trigger fat-burning hormones, but if the adrenals are releasing so much sugar from the tissues and even turning the muscles into sugar, these fat-burning hormones get blocked.

In this state, the body is trying to increase its survival by holding on to fat energy around the vital organs in the stomach area and the face. Of course, the body doesn't seem to care what the person will end up looking like. The face and eyes will become puffy, and a double chin and rounding of the face can develop.

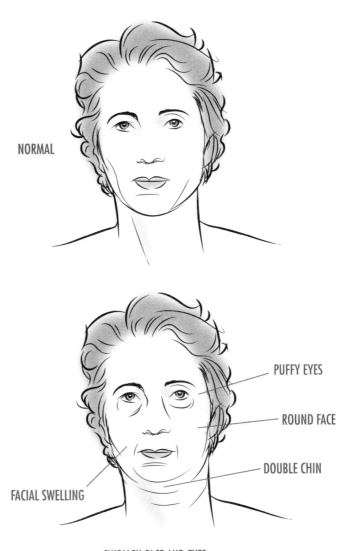

NORMAL

PUFFY EYES

ROUND FACE

DOUBLE CHIN

FACIAL SWELLING

SWOLLEN FACE AND EYES

In order to get into fat burning, there must be NO extra sugar or very limited sugar present in the blood. In the presence of sugar or refined carbohydrates, your body CANNOT and WILL NOT burn fat.[4] So, if the adrenals are constantly releasing sugar, how the heck are you supposed to lose weight?[5] In fact, sugar triggers the fat-storing hormone insulin, which will override all other fat-burning hormones and turn them off. The body will ALWAYS burn sugar in place of fat.

A good thing to do is consume small amounts of protein in between meals to prevent the body from eating itself. Raw nuts and seeds are best. However, if you have a Liver body type, you should not snack between meals except when you are on the Liver Enhancement Plan. The reason for this will be explained further in chapters 8, 9 and 10.

In women, adrenal hormone increases can result in a deeper voice, facial hair and male-pattern hair loss (receding hair line)—but other than that, the person is totally fine! I'm kidding. They can really mess with a woman's body.

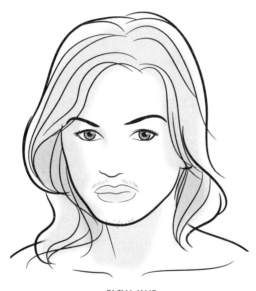

FACIAL HAIR

Acne can occur due to enlargement of the oil glands on the face, especially during women's periods. Atrophy (shrinkage) of the breasts can also be present. The above symptoms are due to an overabundance of male hormone production by the adrenals—androgens (*andro-* means "man").

Both the ovaries and adrenals produce estrogen and testosterone, which when out of balance can influence the oil glands and hair follicles. I have observed if a woman's right ovary is dysfunctional, the left side of her face (cheek) will develop more acne; and if the right ovary is out of balance, the left side of her face will develop more acne—there seems to be a crossover connection.

When excessive adrenal hormones are produced, the person has problems with the mineral calcium. In order to absorb calcium your blood needs to be a certain pH. This term *pH* refers to the acid/alkaline levels. The body has many fluids, which need to be either acid or alkaline. Overproduction of adrenal hormones can increase potassium loss, turning the person's blood pH on the side of too much alkalinity.[6] This prevents calcium from being directed to the bones and muscles, so one gets not only thinning of the bones but muscle cramps in the calves at night. Cramps in the calf muscles come from calcium, magnesium or potassium deficiencies. All three are adrenal problems. I think what's happening is instead of calcium going *into* the body it accumulates *on* the body tissues. I have observed these cases to have a buildup of tartar on their teeth, calcium on the eyes as early cataracts, on the bones as heal spurs, on the joints as arthritis, on the bursas (joint sacs) as bursitis, on the tendons as tendonitis, in the arteries as arteriosclerosis, deposits in the kidneys, and twitching under or on top of the left eyelid.

When the adrenals pump out excess hormones, high levels of calcium are lost through the urine, which is associated with osteoporosis.[7] Without this calcium, a person will have a difficult time getting to sleep, not to mention staying asleep. This is the cause of racing thoughts solving yesterday's problems at 2:00 a.m. when you should be sound asleep.

Leafy green vegetables are the best source of calcium—much better than milk. Pasteurized milk has been heated to a high temperature and, as a result, the calcium is much harder to absorb. A better source of dairy calcium would be plain yogurt or cheese. Yogurt and cheese are fermented and/or cultured products and the friendly cultures and enzymes that are used reorganize amino acids (proteins), making a new food. These new proteins resemble plant proteins and are easier to digest and use by the body.

The adrenal hormones' timing mechanism (clock) controls circadian rhythms—waves of hormones that affect sleep and awake cycles. With adrenal problems everything is backwards; you are tired during the day yet despite being exhausted you can't sleep through the night. The body just won't let you get into the deeper sleep cycles. Because the adrenals counter stress, their production of abnormally high amounts of stress hormones makes it impossible to attain the deep, restful sleep you need to properly rejuvenate the body for the coming day.[8]

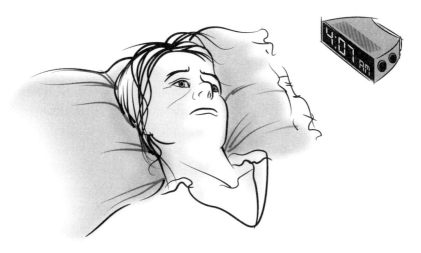

UNABLE TO GET RESTFUL SLEEP AT NIGHT

In the diagram below, you can see normal cortisol (adrenal hormone) levels. Notice that cortisol is supposed to be very minimal during sleep.

CIRCADIAN RHYTHM AND CORTISOL

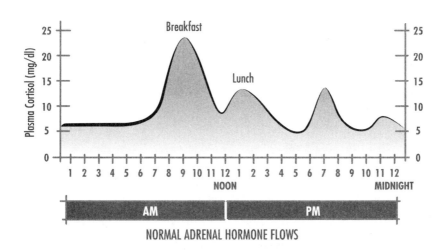

NORMAL ADRENAL HORMONE FLOWS

Certain adrenal hormones are responsible for making you feel awake mentally. Others are responsible for the sleep cycle.

Your body goes through four 90-minute cycles of sleep from superficial to deep. Just imagine trying to sleep while a lion was chasing you. You might be tired but your body would not be. Often a person will just wake up at 2:00–3:00 a.m. for no reason and end up lying there for an hour (or hours) before going back to sleep, if they are lucky. The worst thing about this is not being able to function the next day.

Because everything is backwards, Adrenal types can have bladder issues (leaky bladder, frequent urination) at night even more than during the day.

However, the problem gets worse. Fat-burning effects of certain hormones can occur only during the deep sleep cycles. But with an adrenal problem you are not getting into deep sleep cycles, so the fat-burning effects from exercise can get nullified due to poor sleep.

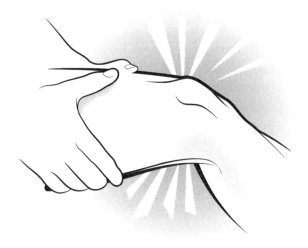

UNRESOLVING PAIN AND INFLAMMATION

Adrenal Deficiency

Exhausted adrenals can cause you to experience pain in different parts of the body because you are running out of anti-inflammatory hormones. If the "on-off switch" within the adrenals gets stuck, a person can go into a chronic stage in which pain and inflammation stay in the body for years. A person can also experience sore muscles that don't seem to recover after exercise. As this situation worsens, fibromyalgia develops, which is a condition of muscle pain throughout the entire body. What happens is there is an excess of inflammation throughout the body's muscles, tendons and connective tissues due to lack of the inflammatory removing hormones normally produced by the adrenal glands. Having pain and inflammation and losing weight don't mix. The stress hormone triggered by the pain can block fat-burning hormones.

As far as muscle tissue is concerned, exercising with weights or doing high-pulse-rate exercise is not a good idea with this condition, since the extra stress overwhelms the adrenals. In chapter 14 you will learn more about the best form of exercise; it involves walking and keeping your pulse rate no higher than 130 beats per minute.

Adrenal exhaustion will also cause overall body exhaustion with an inability to get restful sleep at night. Consequently, the Adrenal type of individual is usually fatigued, dragging their body around during the day, half awake.

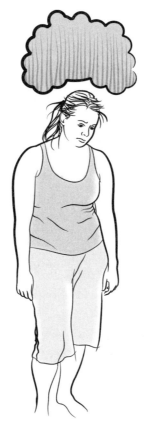

FATIGUED AND DRAGGING THE BODY AROUND

With weak adrenals, the person is more awake in the middle of the night than during the day. They can't get out of bed, feel tired after lunch, feel tired in the early evening, and if they don't get to bed at a certain time, then they can't go to sleep. If the Adrenal type has a sedentary job, they will have a wave of sleepiness right around 2:30–3:00 p.m. Due to a lack of quality sleep, midafternoon naps are desperately needed.

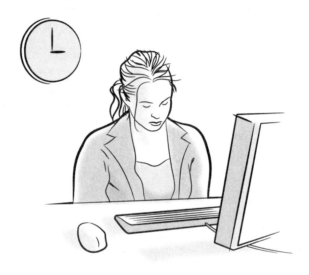

CAN'T STAY AWAKE MIDAFTERNOON

Typically, an individual with burnt-out adrenals has darkened circles under their eyes as well as a very tired appearance. They feel tired, drained and have brain fog. The brain fatigue can greatly affect concentration.

Adrenal types need coffee to wake up — strong Cuban coffee. Europeans use very small cups for coffee; Americans have humongous jugs of coffee. Caffeine—which is also in chocolate, sodas and tea— stimulates adrenal hormones and acts like an artificial energy booster, giving you mental alertness for one or two hours until it wears off. However, over time there are fewer highs and more lows. In college, I would drink pots of coffee at a time, trying to stay up at night and study. At that age most people can get away with it, but at 28 it caught up with me — stomach ulcers, insomnia, inflammation and severe fatigue. Over the years a person can feel depressed and very lethargic from this. Most people don't have depression; they just don't sleep!

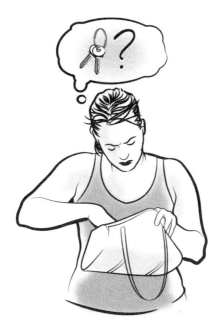

BRAIN FOG OR DULLNESS

Artificial sweeteners also aggravate these hormones. In my last book, I recommended sugar alcohols such as Splenda, xylitol and mannitol as substitutes for sugar. In this book I'm not recommending these at all because they worsen the adrenals. I found a reference saying they can contribute to adrenal tumors in animals. I have discovered that they inhibit weight loss by causing water retention.

An interesting note about tea: Green tea, despite having some caffeine, has anticaffeine properties and tends to not create the same jittery effect that drinking lots of coffee will. In some people it actually helps adrenal function.

If the adrenals do not work properly, this can affect oxygen levels, causing you to feel out of breath, particularly when the body is stressed, such as while climbing stairs.[9] The lower legs also will feel heavier, as if you were carrying around lead ankle weights, especially when you try to exercise on inclined surfaces.

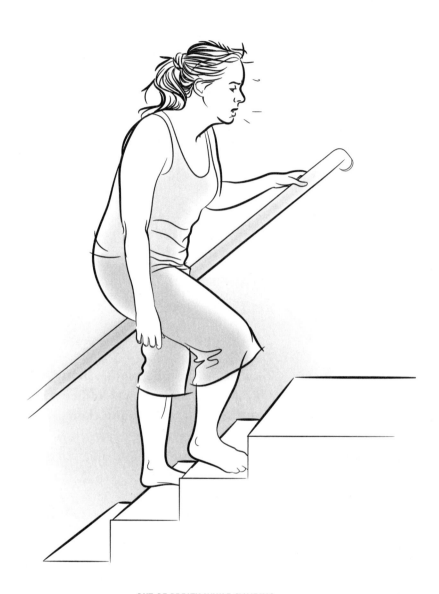

OUT OF BREATH WHILE CLIMBING

The adrenals have another function: controlling blood vessel contraction and relaxation, which affects blood pressure. Adrenal hormones constrict most blood vessels with the exception of two: the vessels in your lungs and the main artery around the heart (coronary). This is why a person with asthma needs a broncho (lung) steroid inhaler (which is adrenal hormones). If the adrenals can't relax the lungs, a constriction and tightening occurs preventing oxygen from entering. The coronary artery, which feeds oxygen to the heart muscle, is also controlled by the adrenal hormone adrenaline. If the adrenals are weak, the coronary can become constricted, especially under stress, preventing blood flow to the heart. This can give tightness in the chest or actual chest pains.

Are you beginning to see the importance of the adrenal glands?

Because the adrenals affect blood vessels, one can have abnormally constricted blood vessels in the inner ear, triggering ringing in the ears or even high blood pressure. High blood pressure could also stem from a calcium buildup in the arteries, since with adrenal problems a person tends to get arteriosclerosis (hardening of the arteries). Initially the top number (systolic) will increase before the bottom number (diastolic).[10]

There is a test called Ragland's in which you take a person's blood pressure lying down and then again standing up. Normally the top number (systolic) should rise 6 to 10 points when you stand up. However, with adrenal stress, the top number will either be lower than 6 points or higher than 10 points. (See illustration on the following page.)

If the person's test result is within normal range and they feel good after exercise, then a more intense workout would be indicated. If it is *not* within normal range and the person feels worse after exercise, then aerobic low-pulse-rate walking exercise would be recommended until the adrenals improve. You can find more on this in chapter 14.

Lie down for 3 to 5 minutes' rest.
Take blood pressure while lying down.

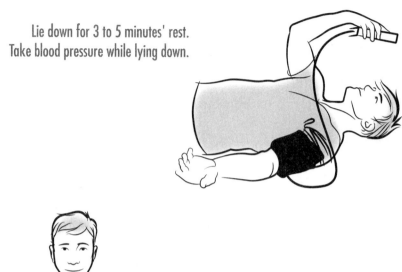

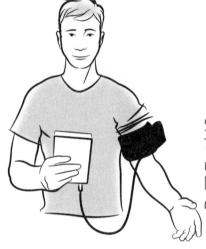

Stand and take blood pressure again.
The top number (systolic) should
normally rise 6 to 10 points. Having a
higher or lower number could mean
adrenal stress.

BLOOD PRESSURE TEST LYING, THEN STANDING

Stress responses to all aspects of life are the hallmark of the adrenals. People who have weak adrenals do not deal well with stress; the littlest things seem to irritate them rather easily. Excessive worry and anxiety are common with adrenal weakness due to the adrenaline stress response (fight or flight).

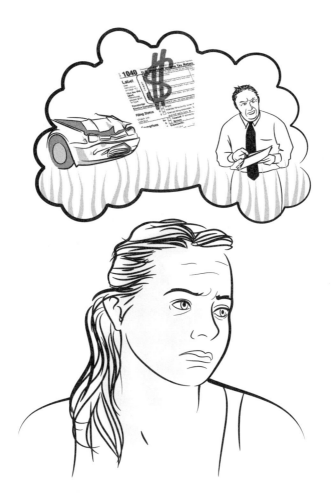

STRESS: EXCESSIVE WORRY AND ANXIETY ARE COMMON

When the adrenals decrease in function, the inability to handle life's stress increases. One patient of mine couldn't even sit through a movie that had any suspense; it would keep her up all night long. I had another patient who didn't have the patience to stand in line at the grocery store.

The adrenal-deficient case is usually worrying 24/7. This is very draining and leads to the need for stimulants — coffee, soda, tea and chocolate. These might give them an hour of clarity or feeling up, but the rest of the day is dull and lacking sharpness. This is the person who is half asleep and who is always visiting their local coffee shop.

Cravings for salt in the form of cheese, pretzels, nuts, popcorn or chips in the evening are common. People search the cupboards late at night for something crunchy and cheesy. This is because the adrenals regulate salts in the body.

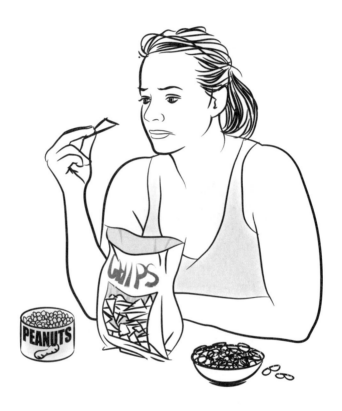

CRAVINGS FOR SALT OR CHEESE AT NIGHT

With salt and mineral imbalances, fluids can get out of balance, causing the individual to retain fluid (outside the cells) yet be dehydrated (inside the cells) at the same time.

Wherever sodium goes, water will accumulate. So when sodium gets lost through the urine, dehydration can occur. Often, drinking more water does not hydrate the person because there is too little sodium to balance it. In fact, I have found that people who drink the most water have the greatest dehydration.

FYI (for your information): Never consume table salt; use good quality sea salt. Sea salt has 84 minerals and table salt has only 2.

There is definitely a huge push for everyone to drink more water. Drinking more water so that you'll eat less usually won't satisfy you for more than 45 seconds. Instead it will make you feel bloated and cause you to get up several times during the night to use the bathroom, not to mention creating those little rings around your lower legs and ankles when you take off your socks at night.

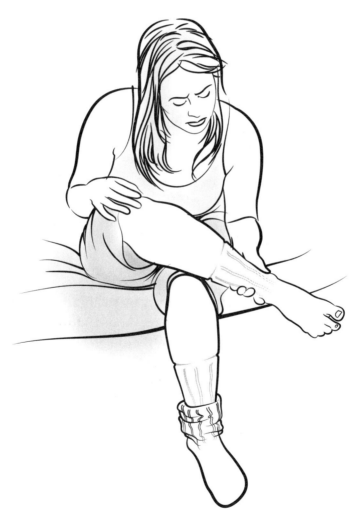

ANKLES SWELLING AT NIGHT

Many people make the mistake of drinking large quantities of water. I don't know who started the rumor that you need 8 to 10 glasses of water per day, or a gallon of ice-cold water — maybe the bottled-water companies. But if you drink too much of it, you can flush out minerals that are holding the water there in the first place, creating even more of an imbalance.

People use the same logic as they do for fat: If you are fat, you need to avoid fat calories; therefore, if your body is made mostly of water, then you need to drink water. Neither of these statements is true. In regard to fat calories, you have to understand that the hormones look at food differently. And with water, you should drink it only when you are thirsty. Don't ever force yourself to drink water — drink when you are thirsty!

FYI: Drinking water doesn't flush out fat.

A deficiency of adrenal hormones can also create cravings for chocolate. This is because some of the body's serotonin is produced by the adrenal glands. Serotonin creates a sense of well-being or comfort, and chocolate stimulates serotonin. People who crave chocolate are really craving the adrenal hormone serotonin.

If you take the combination of salt and chocolate, you get chocolate-covered pretzels. In fact, this is how I diagnose adrenal problems — I simply hold up a chocolate-covered pretzel in front of a person's face and see if they go for it.

The adrenals affect blood sugar levels.[11] So, poor adrenal function could cause the person to experience sugar cravings in addition to salt and chocolate cravings during the late afternoons and evenings.

In the following chart, you can see the different symptoms of high blood sugar and low blood sugar. High blood sugar (such as after a Thanksgiving meal) can produce brain fog, and low blood sugar (from skipping a meal) can also produce brain fog, as well as anxiety and even cravings for sweets.

BRAIN FOG AND FATIGUE	NEED A NAP (EYES TIRED)

140
120
100
80
70
60

HIGH BLOOD SUGAR

FEELING YOUR BEST

LOW BLOOD SUGAR

SUGAR CRAVING

SUGAR CRAVING

ANXIETY, DEPRESSION, MOODY, IRRITABLE, SUGAR CRAVING

8:00 a.m.   10:00 a.m.   NOON   2:00 p.m.   4:00 p.m.   6:00 p.m.   8:00 p.m.

FACTS ABOUT BLOOD SUGAR

SKIPPED MEAL (BREAKFAST) TRIGGERS LOW BLOOD SUGAR LEVELS

LETTING YOURSELF GET HUNGRY BETWEEN MEALS DROPS BLOOD SUGAR LEVELS

EATING A HIGH-CARBOHYDRATE BREAKFAST CREATES LOW BLOOD SUGAR LEVELS, TRIGGERING CRAVINGS LATE AFTERNOON AND LATE NIGHT

OVEREATING ALSO TRIGGERS HIGH BLOOD SUGAR LEVELS AND INSULIN RESPONSE

Your body will tell you what deficiency you have, based on what you crave. If you crave cheese or salt, this could mean you are low in sodium and your adrenal hormones are too low. If you crave grapefruit or melon, it could mean you're low in potassium and your adrenal hormones are too high. Craving licorice could indicate you are deficient in another adrenal hormone. The program I'm about to recommend will assist in giving the body what it needs so that you don't crave the wrong foods.

> FYI: Children who eat dirt or clay, or women who chew on ice during pregnancy, could be deficient in iron. (I would recommend eating beets instead of dirt.) Craving ice cream or cheese could also mean you are low in calcium, which indicates an adrenal problem.

Since the adrenal glands affect the immune system to a large degree, weakened adrenals can also cause increased susceptibility to viruses. Adrenal hormones suppress immune responses — such as inflammation, and itching of hives from excess histamine — as well as infections, viruses, etc. This is why when someone takes a steroid like prednisone — which is an adrenal hormone — the allergic reaction, asthma or even inflammation from poison ivy can disappear.[12] Allergies, asthma and chemical sensitivities occur in a body with weakened adrenals. This is the reason a person who experiences a severe allergy reaction (anaphylactic shock) needs what is called an EpiPen. An EpiPen is epinephrine (also known as adrenaline), which is a main hormone of the adrenals, in an injectable form.

> FYI: Viruses cannot be killed because they are not alive in the first place. Viruses are pieces of genetic material wrapped in a sac— that's all. But once inside your body, a weak cell can allow them to enter. When the virus enters your cell, it combines with your DNA and starts replicating. It's like a copy machine gone out of control, destroying your cells. A virus is so small that it would compare in size to a ping-pong ball if a bacteria were the size of the Empire State Building. It could fit through the pores of a porcelain dish. Viruses enter your body and never leave. They go into remission or hiding. Don't ever believe anyone who tells you to take some medication to kill the virus—it won't. Viruses can travel through the body into the spinal cord or brain and stay there. They are like seeds in the ground, waiting for the right environment. They wait for your resistance to be lowered so they can kick you when you are weak.

> The best defense against viruses, especially the flu, is to keep your resistance high by ensuring your adrenals are strong.

When the immune system goes crazy and starts to attack your own cells — autoimmune (self-attack) — the adrenal hormones are not doing their job. Normally, adrenal hormones are supposed to suppress immune cells. When this suppress function is broken, the immune system can go out of control.

The adrenals can overwork and underwork. Depending on the state they are in, you will experience different symptoms. I have frequently observed that a person will start with their adrenals in overdrive due to stress, then burn them out into an underworking adrenal situation. But it's not always that cut and dried, as a person might have a combination of symptoms. The eating and exercising program is designed to help normalize either overworking or underworking adrenals. Due to the destructive nature of the adrenals on your muscles, you'll be modifying the Liver Enhancement by adding more protein.

Causes of the Adrenal Body Type

There are several things that worsen or burn out the adrenal glands. The biggest of these is taking adrenal hormones; this could be in the form of prednisone or steroids (same thing). When you bypass the body and give it straight hormones, the adrenals don't have to produce their own. As a side effect this severely weakens the adrenals. I'm not recommending avoiding steroids if your doctor has advised them. I had a patient who was a swimsuit model; she developed a heel spur and received a steroid injection for pain. Four years later she developed a huge midsection with lots of stubborn weight. Steroids tend to make you put on weight by affecting the adrenals.

The second cause of adrenal problems comes from taking too much synthetic ascorbic acid (known as vitamin C). In nature, vitamin C comes in a whole-complex form, consisting of ascorbic acid, vitamin P factors (bioflavonoids), vitamin K and J factors, organic copper and the enzyme tyrosinase. The ascorbic acid antioxidant element is only one part. Taking this one part in huge doses can severely aggravate the adrenals, since the adrenal glands are a storage system for vitamin C. Man-made vitamin C (ascorbic acid) is often produced from cornstarch and sulfuric acid. You could even feel good taking these synthetics for a while, because they act as a stimulant. However, I've had patients take grams (one gram is 1,000 milligrams) of the stuff and end up with adrenal problems down the road. Always take vitamin C in its whole form from food. In its whole form you rarely see the ascorbic acid part over 100 milligrams.

The third cause of weak adrenals is overwhelming stress to the body. Years of not sleeping, living with stressful people, a stressful environment, experiencing the loss of a loved one, going through a divorce, etc., can drain the adrenal glands.

The fourth cause of trouble with the adrenal glands is infection, especially from fungus, unfriendly yeast and viruses. The adrenals get a major amount of blood flow because they are above the kidneys. These microbes travel through the blood and get trapped in the adrenals and create problems later in life.

The fifth source of adrenal problems stems from a combination of taking stimulants and having nutritional deficiencies. Stimulants include caffeine, appetite suppressors, sugar, nicotine, synthetic vitamins, herbal stimulants (ma huang) and drugs. These items deplete vitamins (mainly B vitamins) and minerals (particularly potassium and calcium). Add in poor eating habits and lots of refined sugars and grains and you can end up with exhausted adrenals.

The following are symptoms the Adrenal type can experience from poorly working adrenal glands.

Adrenal Type Symptoms

- Pendulous abdomen (sagging and hanging)
- Midsection weight
- Buffalo hump (fat pad) at the upper back, lower neck area
- Thinner legs and arms
- Weakness
- Fatigue
- Lethargy
- Depression
- Sleepiness
- Insomnia
- Difficulty getting out of bed in the morning
- Need for midafternoon naps
- Nervousness
- Anxiety (worry); frequent feelings of stress
- Can't tolerate stress
- Thinning skin
- Acne or poor skin
- May have white or discolored patches on skin
- Reddish purple stretch marks on the stomach, thighs, buttocks, arms and breasts
- Red cheeks
- Round or moon face
- Puffy face and eyes
- Dark circles around eyes
- Double chin
- Facial hair
- Full eyebrows
- Receding hairline
- Deeper voice
- Sparse hair on forearms and lower legs
- Atrophy of breasts
- Tightness in chest, or chest pains
- High blood pressure
- Lax ligaments—weak ankles and knees
- Weak or brittle bones (due to a loss of calcium and protein)

- Difficulty absorbing calcium
- Needs coffee to wake up
- Salt, cheese, chocolate and sugar cravings, late afternoon and evening
- Inflammation or pain in joints, back, neck
- Heel spurs
- Overreactive immune system — allergies, chemical sensitivities
- Autoimmune conditions
- Fibromyalgia
- Asthma
- Increased susceptibility to viruses
- Dehydrated (intracellular) despite amount of water drunk
- Fluid retention in between cells
- Pitting edema (especially in ankles)
- Gets out of breath when climbing stairs
- Legs feel heavy, especially when exercising
- Moodiness and irritability
- Brain fog or dullness
- Ringing in ears
- Low sex drive

6

The Ovary Type

The Ovaries

The ovaries produce three hormones responsible for controlling the menstrual cycle. They release eggs every month and are in charge of making the environment suitable for the eggs' growth. One of these hormones is estrogen. It creates the fat layer around a female body, specifically around the ovaries — hips, buttocks and lower abdomen.

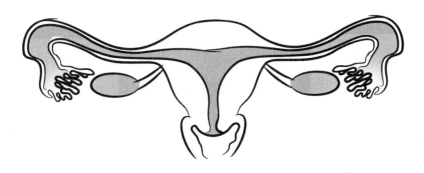

THE OVARIES

The Ovary Type

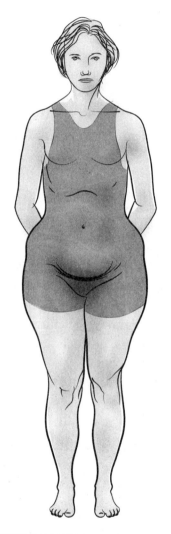

LOWER BODY WEIGHT—"SADDLEBAGS"

The following is a description of what happens when the ovaries don't function properly.

When ovaries become dysfunctional, they can produce an excess of estrogen, which causes more fat. I have observed that this fat is deposited on "saddlebag" thighs, the lower stomach and the buttocks. The lower stomach fat usually shows up just below the bellybutton as a bulge.

Fat cells, by the way, also produce estrogen.

Problems that can be caused by the ovaries include PMS (premenstrual syndrome), cravings at certain times of the month, bloating at certain times of the month, extra painful cramps and excessive menstrual bleeding, as well as depression during the menstrual cycle. Apart from that, there is no problem at all!

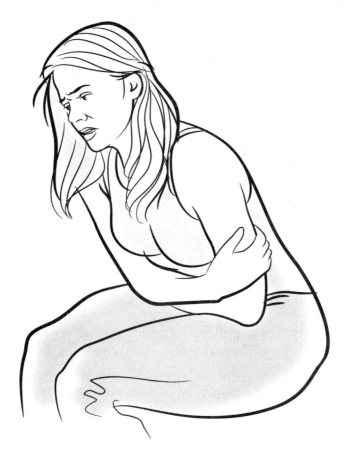

EXTRA PAINFUL CRAMPS

Many times a person with an Ovary body type experiences pain on either side of their lower-back area. Pain can also be in one of the knees, as the pain is being referred from one of the ovaries.

The pictures below show the changes from a normal body shape through the progressive stages of the Ovary type.

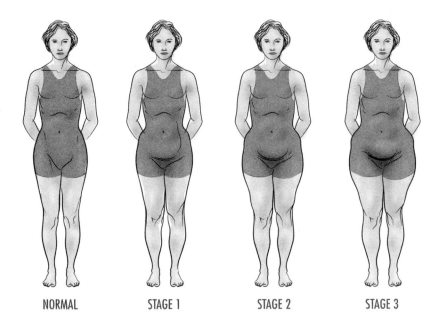

NORMAL   STAGE 1   STAGE 2   STAGE 3

Causes of the Ovary Body Type

Ovaries are very sensitive to environmental hormones. Environmental hormones are those that come from birth control pills, hormone replacement therapy (HRT) and other external supplies of hormones that enter the body. Growth hormones fed to beef, poultry and farm-raised fish are in this category. Chemicals that mimic hormones, such as pesticides and DDT, also affect the ovaries, uterus and breasts. Because the ovaries produce estrogen, when these external estrogens not produced by the body enter the system, the ovaries' own production becomes disrupted.

This can create one of two situations:

- The ovaries increase their production of estrogen, creating more fat deposits around the hips, thighs and lower stomach.

- The ovaries shut down their production of estrogen. When this happens, a part of the brain has to overcompensate and increase its hormone messages for the ovaries to produce more hormones. This is similar to a boss finding an employee not doing his job; he might then begin to put pressure on this individual to get back to work!

This second scenario is what can cause ovarian cysts and other growths. These cysts can make the affected ovary produce even more estrogen, resulting in additional fat around your thighs and hips. Pesticides on our foods can also act like estrogen and cause cysts, fibroids (fibrous growths) and tumors on the ovaries and uterus. They can create the same effect as environmental estrogens.

When a woman produces extra estrogen, the thyroid can get blocked. Anytime estrogen increases, as in pregnancy, the thyroid hormones are inhibited. The person might go to the doctor and have her thyroid checked, yet it isn't bad enough to show as being abnormal. A good endocrinologist will assess the entire endocrine system, including ovarian function.

It only takes very small amounts of estrogen and chemicals to create these effects; but by cleaning from the diet things that mimic estrogen, one can assist in bringing these hormones and glands back into a normal balance. For the Ovary type it is important to consume organic, hormone-free foods as much as possible.

The Menopause Backup Organ

During menopause the ovaries shut down. When this occurs the adrenal glands kick in and begin producing hormones similar to those the ovaries once produced, only in smaller quantities because the woman will not be giving birth. This fact is rarely known by the layperson. If the adrenal glands are weak or sluggish during menopause, they cannot act as the ovaries' backup organ and a person will usually start to have problems such as weight gain, hot flashes, night sweats and vaginal dryness.

A small part of the brain controls the ovaries. It is located right next to the temperature control center that affects perspiration, heart rate and sweating. When the ovaries shut down during menopause, if the adrenals cannot act as the backup the way they're supposed to, stress is placed on the controlling part of the brain. The lack of return communication from the adrenals to the brain creates stress in the perspiration center, causing a flush of heat and sweating. It could be likened to talking to or asking a question of your spouse while he or she is not responding to you. Being ignored would eventually upset you. In a similar way, your body reacts in the form of stress at the temperature center in the brain, which creates a flood of heat at any time of the day or night. That is what hot flashes are. Someone's trying to talk, but no one is listening.

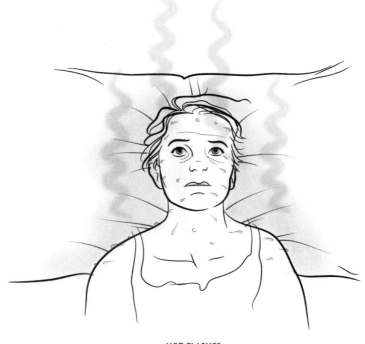

HOT FLASHES

The reason why HRT often helps with hot flashes is because it gives the brain a return message — the answer it is waiting for — thus calming everything down. It's an artificial reply but it completes the circuit and turns off the heat. The only problem with this situation is some slight minor adverse complications seven years down the road — such as *strokes, heart disease, cancer* and *tumors of the liver.* Apart from that, it's totally safe!

I've observed that before age 52 the person might have a thinner waist with an Ovary body shape; then after age 52 she starts looking like an Adrenal shape (belly fat). This is because the adrenal gland is the backup to the ovaries.

Below is a list of symptoms the Ovary type can experience from improperly working ovaries.

Ovary Type Symptoms

- Weight gain in hips, thighs and buttocks, with a lower stomach bulge
- History of PMS
- Weight gain or bloating around that time of the month
- Ovarian cysts
- Cyclic fatigue
- Cyclic brain fog
- Cyclic pain in the lower back or hips
- Cyclic pain in the knee
- Cyclic lack of libido
- Infertility
- Hot flashes
- Night sweats
- Vaginal dryness
- Cyclic acne
- Cyclic mood swings
- Extra painful cramps
- Excessive menstrual bleeding
- Cyclic constipation
- Cyclic thinning of the hair
- Depression during menstrual cycle
- Cravings at certain times of the month

7

The Thyroid Type

The Thyroid Gland

Located in the lower part of the neck, and approximately 2½ inches wide, the thyroid gland regulates the rate at which the body burns food and controls the production of certain body tissues such as nails and hair. The thyroid gland also regulates body temperature, breakdown of carbohydrates, mental clarity and well-being, energy levels and even vitamin absorption. Cholesterol levels, hair texture, nail strength, suppleness or dryness of the skin and sex drive are all directly influenced by the thyroid.

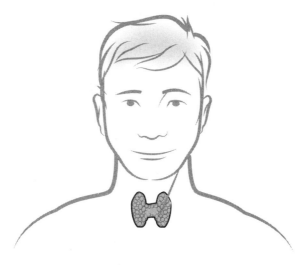

THE THYROID GLAND

The thyroid gland releases a combination of several different hormones. Their names aren't as important as their purpose — to speed up the metabolism of the body.

Metabolism refers to the rate or speed at which, or the degree to which, the body breaks down food and changes it into living tissue and energy. *Metabolism* also has a subdefinition, "the releasing of energy (burning of fat) from fat cells." And your metabolism is controlled by hormones.

The Thyroid Type

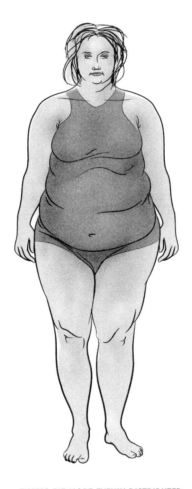

EXCESS FAT MORE EVENLY DISTRIBUTED

The Sluggish Thyroid

The first major consequence of a sluggish thyroid is a slow metabolism. Everything is slower. Brain processes can be suppressed, triggering depression, lethargy and a general apathetic feeling.

A loss of libido (sex drive) can occur with a slow thyroid. It could also cause a complete loss of the menstrual cycle.

Another manifestation is a feeling of being tired all the time, despite sleeping for long hours. This is chronic fatigue. Its distinct feature is feeling more awake in the morning but ready for bed at 8:00 p.m. The thyroid also controls the oil glands and blood flow to the skin. A sluggish thyroid can mean dry skin and dry, brittle hair. With a thyroid problem, a person could attempt to curl her hair and not be able to maintain the curl. She might even lose the outer third of her eyebrows.

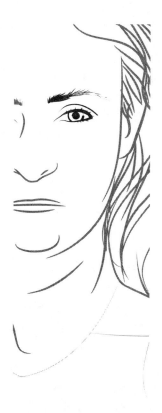

LOSS OF THE OUTER EYEBROWS

Since the thyroid gland controls metabolism, in a nonoptimum state it begins to drive body temperature to well below normal, causing cold hands and feet. Sufferers need to wear extra clothing, even in moderate climates. Some people have to wear socks to bed. What's interesting is I've never met a person with cold feet who didn't have a spouse with warm feet — I guess opposites attract.

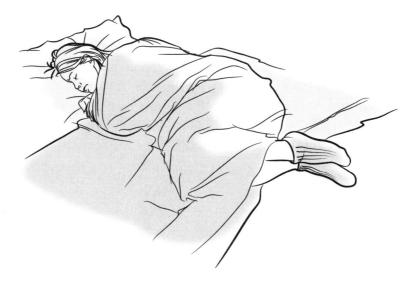

NEEDS TO WEAR SOCKS TO BED AT NIGHT

Because everything is slower, the body will demand quick energy as in carbohydrate cravings. The most common cravings I have observed with the Thyroid type are starches, especially bread, and in particular sourdough bread just out of the oven with some butter.

I had this guy tell me that he didn't eat carbohydrates. I said, "Okay, what did you eat for breakfast?" He replied, "Apple pie from McDonald's." I told him, "That is carbohydrate." He said, "No it's not; it's apples."

There seems to be some confusion about what a carbohydrate is, so let me define it. A carbohydrate is any of a group of substances made of carbon, hydrogen and oxygen, including the sugars and starches. There are several types of carbohydrates: grains, vegetables, fruits and sugars. Unrefined carbohydrates provide vitamins and minerals as well as fiber, whereas refined grains have little nutrient value. Vegetable starches such as potatoes, yams, corn, French fries and hash browns are easily converted to fat, and some of the sweeter fruits have a greater effect on insulin. I will go over this in more detail in chapter 9.

The carbohydrates we are primarily concerned about are those that have been refined. Breads, pasta, cereals, crackers, pancakes, waffles, donuts, cakes, muffins, rice cakes, cookies, candy, chocolate, juice, alcohol, wine, beer and ice cream are all refined carbohydrates. And Thyroid types can crave any of these.

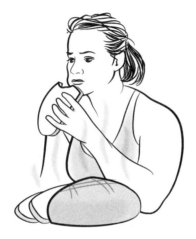

CRAVINGS FOR BREAD

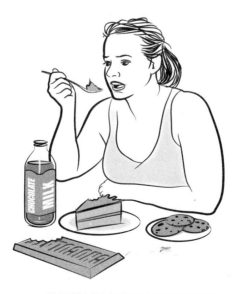

CRAVINGS FOR SUGARY CARBOHYDRATES

Have you ever eaten something that you knew you shouldn't have—at least once in your life? What have you normally said to justify it? "I deserve it." "I'll work out twice as hard tomorrow." "You have to die from something; might as well enjoy yourself." "If I eat it up, it won't be in the house to tempt me." "It doesn't count if no one sees me." "It's a holiday." "They wouldn't make it if it wasn't okay to eat"—or, my favorite, "Everything in moderation."

The main problem with burning fat is this: in the presence of refined carbohydrates (especially sugar), your body cannot burn fat. I'm sorry! And to top it off, the excess carbohydrate is converted into fat and cholesterol.[1]

High Cholesterol

Are You Sure It's Really Genetics or Eating Fatty Foods?

There are rare genetic disorders characterized by an accumulation of large quantities of fat in the blood. If they're rare, how do you explain the millions of people who have high cholesterol? Some people will even tell you it's bad genes and you should have picked your parents more wisely. Good luck! And what about eating fat—does that cause high cholesterol? If that is true, then how do you explain why a person still needs cholesterol medication despite having cut all the fat out of their diet? There is another condition called familial hypercholesterolemia (excessive cholesterol in the blood), which shows up in seven out of a thousand people. So, rather than accept someone's opinion on whether you have a genetic cholesterol problem, get evaluated to find out the facts. The point is, if your thyroid is not working correctly, your cholesterol could be high in spite of what you are eating and all your efforts to keep it low.

> Did you know that 75 percent of the cholesterol in your body is made by your body? Cholesterol is required by the body to make hormones.

The need for vitamins greatly increases with a thyroid weakness. The weakness means the vitamins are just not absorbed. The body dumps them through the urine—expensive urine because these vitamins are wasted. Such people are usually taking vitamin supplements and not feeling any different.

> By the way, what was the first vitamin that was ever discovered? Was it C? No. How about D? No. The answer is A. Then came B, then C, then D and E.

The body-fat pattern resulting from a sluggish thyroid is an overall fat distribution. The pictures below show the changes from a normal body shape through the progressive stages of the Thyroid type.

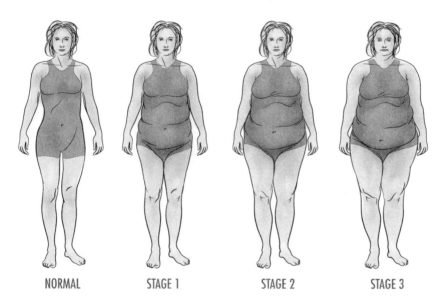

| NORMAL | STAGE 1 | STAGE 2 | STAGE 3 |

As a side note, a person with a true sluggish thyroid problem is not solely retaining fat. They have a great deal of waste-like-fluid weight that contributes to the appearance of having an overall excess weight problem. As mentioned in chapter 2, this condition is called myxedema and is the result of a thyroid that is not working to full capacity.

Many people think they have attention deficit disorder (ADD) when in fact they may have a weak thyroid. Have you ever known people who walked into a room and forgot why? Have you ever talked to someone you could tell was a bit checked out? This type of lethargy can be attributed to poor thyroid function. And without really spending the time to evaluate and find the true cause, a person could be put on Ritalin by mistake.

> I really think the problem with our healthcare system narrows down to incomplete evaluation. If you have pain, you are given a pill; high blood pressure—pill; high cholesterol—pill; ADD—pill. This is what I call duct-tape therapy. There is very little discovery of underlying causes to these problems. If it were HEALTHcare it would work; but it's disease care. There's hardly any prevention or food therapy. Even worse is the lazy diagnosis—you know, "You're getting older now and you have to accept the fact that these things come with age." Or, "It's your genetics; you have the fat gene." Or, "You're African American and at risk for ____, so take these pills the rest of your life." Everything is heavy on treatment but very light on prevention or evaluation to find the real cause.

The skin, hair and nails are all made up of body protein, which becomes altered when the thyroid can no longer do its job. A person with a thyroid problem can have trouble with hair loss or thinning hair.

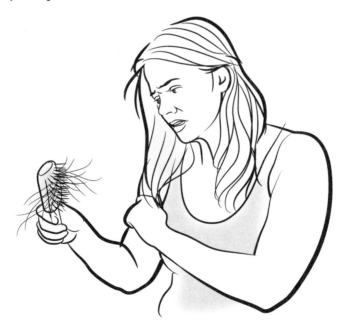

HAIR LOSS OR THINNING HAIR

Sagging skin under the arms, chin or midsection can occur because the body protein that holds the skin firm is breaking down faster than it is building up. Have you ever met someone with these symptoms — a friend, neighbor, relative or co-worker?

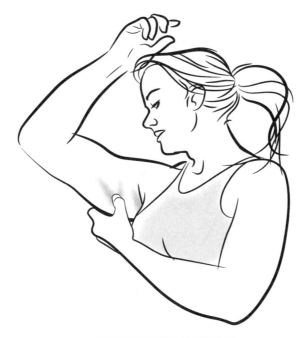

LOOSE SKIN UNDER UPPER ARMS

Your nails especially are made from protein, and because the person's body protein is breaking down faster than it can be built up, the fingernails can become brittle with prominent vertical (up-and-down) ridges.

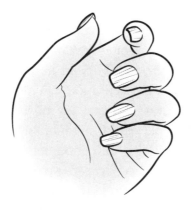

VERTICAL RIDGES ON THE NAILS

A poorly functioning thyroid gland produces puffiness around the eyes and sagging of the eyelids. If it's bad enough, the tongue even thickens, causing a slight slurring of speech, and the voice can become deeper and rougher in sound. The tongue can develop little dished indentations on the sides; it is getting bigger and is being shaped by the inside of the teeth.

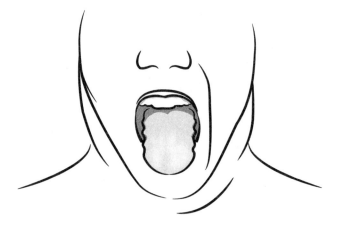

INDENTATIONS ON SIDES OF TONGUE

Glands Work with Each Other

To complicate things, all the glands interact with one another, and we earlier looked at some of these relationships. In regard to the thyroid gland, if the ovaries overproduce estrogen, the thyroid will decrease in function as a secondary problem. This is why women notice weight gain and even a sluggish thyroid after pregnancy, or after taking birth control pills or being on hormone replacement therapy. Thyroid hormones can interfere with the adrenal hormones. Their inactivation can then signal the brain to direct the production of more adrenal hormones through its feedback mechanism.[2] And since 80 percent of thyroid function occurs through the liver, without the liver working well a good portion of thyroid hormone activation can be inhibited. In fact, if the liver is damaged, the main thyroid hormone will not be broken down, leading to excess thyroid hormone in the blood. These are two reasons why you will begin this program with the Liver Enhancement Plan.

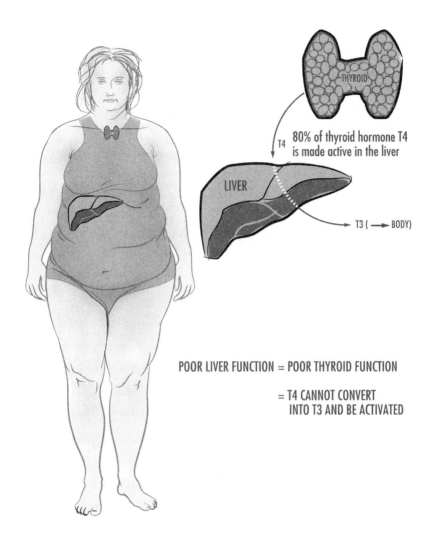

T4   80% of thyroid hormone T4 is made active in the liver

THYROID

LIVER

T3 (⟶ BODY)

POOR LIVER FUNCTION = POOR THYROID FUNCTION

= T4 CANNOT CONVERT
INTO T3 AND BE ACTIVATED

Causes of the Thyroid Body Type

Some medical journals say that the fundamental cause of a sluggish thyroid is a *deficiency* of thyroid hormones, which control metabolism. But the question that should be asked is, WHY is there a deficiency of these hormones in the first place?

There is accumulating information today that toxic environmental factors, such as estrogen mimics, can be linked to thyroid deficiencies.

Scientists who study poisons in the environment are finding this connection. The following are a couple of examples of what is being discovered.

> In his book *What Your Doctor May Not Tell You about Menopause*, Dr. John Lee states: "My hypothesis is that estrogen inhibits thyroid action in the cells, probably interfering with the binding of thyroid to its receptor" [part of the cell that connects with hormones].[3]

> Mary Shomon writes in her book *Living Well with Hypothyroidism*: "Hypothyroidism [low thyroid] is sometimes considered a symptom of estrogen dominance."[4]

Past infections can be a factor with the Thyroid type. The virus that causes Mono (kissing disease), also known as Epstein-Barr virus (EBV), can sometimes affect thyroid function later in life. Other viruses and even bacteria can influence the thyroid.

Injuries to the thyroid from being hit in the neck—an example being a seat belt injury from an auto accident—can influence thyroid function. I knew of a patient who had played baseball and a ball had hit her in the lower throat. Several years later, she ended up with a thyroid problem.

I had another patient who developed thyroid disease after being exposed to radiation. This was the 1986 Chernobyl accident (radioactive fallout) in Ukraine.

Your own ovaries could be causing your thyroid problem (unless you're a man, of course). A cyst or fibroid on the ovary can produce excessive estrogen in the body. This includes polycystic ovarian syndrome (PCOS)—a condition where multiple small cysts form in the ovaries (*poly* means "many"), related to the ovary's failure to release an egg. PCOS can create facial hair, weight gain, insulin resistance and a disruption in the menstrual cycle. So, there could be primary ovarian problems causing a secondary thyroid problem. This could trigger thyroid symptoms, yet the true problem would be the ovaries.

> FYI: If you have PCOS, I would recommend avoiding all estrogen triggers—hormones in our food supply, soy products, and foods that have been sprayed with pesticides; consume organic produce as much as possible. One of my female patients always had a flare-up of cysts when she ate commercial ice cream, which contained extra hormones and chemicals.

Another activity that inhibits thyroid hormones is low-calorie diets. When you fast or cut calories, your thyroid compensates by lowering the metabolic rate. This is a survival way of adapting to less food. That is why it's crucial to never again restrict calories and to not let yourself get hungry.

Estrogen

Estrogen inhibits thyroid function.

Some women develop thyroid problems after pregnancy due to the high levels of estrogen produced; and if a woman who has a thyroid weakness goes through pregnancy, her thyroid medication will usually need to be increased.

These statements raise two key questions: If estrogen inhibits thyroid function, then how are we being exposed to increased amounts of estrogen? And how much estrogen exposure does an average person get on a daily basis?

Estrogen is the number one hormone added to the feed of animals we consume. It is fed to cattle, turkeys, chickens and farm-raised fish. This hormone makes these animals grow faster and plumper. It is more costly, for example, to grow hormone-free chickens for 22 weeks than to grow hormone-fed chickens for only 6 weeks. I believe out of all the things that go into your body, commercial milk contains the highest amount of estrogen. Always drink organic milk, if you're going to drink it at all.

Most European countries do not use growth hormones on their animals and some refuse to buy American hormone-fed meats. Could this be why Americans are fatter?

A common argument against this concept is that the hormone amounts given to animals are so small they have no effect upon the body. But there is far too much evidence available that supports the effects of estrogen. It takes very minute amounts of estrogen in the body to create effects.[6] And pesticides, insecticides, DDT and many other chemicals mimic estrogen in the body, adversely affecting the thyroid.

Another common argument is, if these chemicals are this damaging to our hormones, why doesn't the Environmental Protection Agency advise the public of the thyroid-chemical connection? The reason is that there is a long delay time between exposure and showing symptoms, which makes it hard to pinpoint the actual cause. It could take more than 30 years.

If you have a Thyroid body type, I highly recommend you reduce your dietary food exposure to estrogen by eliminating foods that contain growth hormones. It would also help to reduce the consumption of chemicals (pesticides, insecticides, DDT, etc.) that mimic this hormone, by either introducing organic foods into your diet or at least scrubbing your fruits and vegetables before eating them.

Red wine unfortunately has estrogen-like compounds. I would advise cutting back to no more than two bottles a night — I'm just kidding. You need to avoid all alcohol on this program. Come on, we need to give your liver a break! I know what you are saying — you drink it for health reasons, right?

Cruciferous Vegetables and Iodine

Cruciferous vegetables, which belong to the cabbage family, include kale, radishes, Brussels sprouts, cabbage, bok choy, etc. — you know, the foods that people normally never eat. Cruciferous vegetables are anti-iodine, meaning they tend to deplete iodine, which the thyroid needs in order to function.[5] When I say "tend to deplete iodine," I mean very slightly. You would have to eat ALL cruciferous and nothing else to create this effect. Most of the other foods you eat put the iodine right back, so I wouldn't be too concerned. But if you feel unsure about this and want to eat cruciferous vegetables, just take some extra iodine — sea kelp, dulse or alfalfa — and go ahead and receive the benefits of these vegetables, because they are also antiestrogen foods. I believe their benefits far outweigh any liability.

The following are symptoms the Thyroid type can experience from a poorly working thyroid gland.

Thyroid Type Symptoms

- Weakness
- Fatigue
- Lethargy
- Sleepiness
- Need for midafternoon naps
- Generalized weight gain
- Sagging skin under arms, chin or midsection
- Low/poor appetite
- Craving bread, pasta, chocolate, sweets
- High cholesterol
- Brittle nails with vertical ridges
- Hair stiff and dry
- Hair loss or thinning hair
- Dry skin
- Puffiness around eyes
- Sagging eyelids
- Outer eyebrows thinning or absent
- Slight rosiness or reddening of the face
- Poor short-term memory and focus
- Depression
- Apathetic (loss of hope)
- Difficulty making decisions
- Low body temperature
- Cold intolerance (need to put on a sweater or more covers while sleeping)
- Cold feet and/or hands
- Loss of libido
- Loss of menstrual cycle
- Indentations on sides of tongue
- Thickening of tongue
- Voice deeper and rougher in sound

8

The Liver Type

The Liver

The liver is the body's filtration system. It filters out microbes, drugs and dead cells from the body as an immune function. Every hormone, chemical, bacteria, virus, fungus and parasite is filtered through the liver. It is similar to an oil filter in your car. In addition, it acts as a digestive organ, breaking down fats, proteins and even carbohydrates. It can also make sugar out of protein.

The liver is a major organ for detoxification; it works to break down the chemicals taken in from toxins on foods to which you are exposed daily. It uses sulfur to break down toxic chemicals into harmless ones. Eggs, cruciferous vegetables (e.g., broccoli, cabbage, Brussels sprouts, cauliflower and kale), raw garlic and onions are rich sources of sulfur.

Cruciferous vegetables have some unique properties, including being antiestrogenic and anticarcinogenic (anticancer causing); and since many hormone problems stem from excessive estrogen and toxins, it would be wise to eat as many of these vegetables as possible. In fact, they are the central food for a Liver type.

When the liver gets damaged over the years, toxins that are normally filtered out can recirculate through the body, re-exposing delicate glands to harmful compounds, triggering a toxic overload. Synthetic estrogen from growth hormones, medications, aspirin, birth control pills and

HRT (hormone replacement therapy) also causes huge side effects of damage to the liver.

The liver has over five hundred known functions and every fat-burning hormone works through the liver. This is why our program starts with the Liver Enhancement Plan.

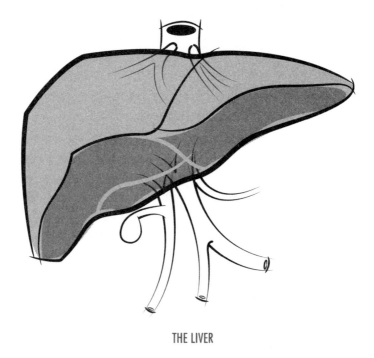

THE LIVER

The following is a description of what happens when the liver does not function properly.

When damaged, the liver causes a potbelly appearance. This protruding abdomen is not always fat; it could be fluid. If the liver is not functioning well it can leak fluid into the stomach area within the abdomen. This characteristic is called *ascites*, which comes from the Greek *askos*, meaning "bladder," "belly" or "wineskin" (animal skin used to hold wine). If you push the stomach from side to side, it looks and feels like a water balloon. An ultrasound is the best way to confirm fluid in the abdomen.

The Liver Type

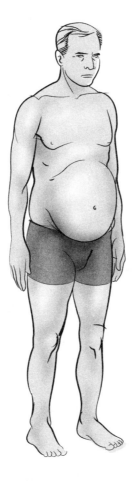

PROTRUDING STOMACH—POTBELLY

Have you ever seen the skinny guy with a potbelly on the beach wearing a Speedo? Sorry for the image. One female patient told me, "Yes, I think I've seen this person before . . . every night before I go to bed!" That is ascites—water weight in the abdomen. There is a sac inside the abdomen area that fills up as the improperly working liver leaks liquid. The fluid is leaking because the liver is not able to produce proteins—it's a low-protein situation that can't be fixed by just eating more protein. You can only improve this by eating high-quality proteins and lots of vegetables that take the stress off the liver and let it heal. This has also been called a "beer gut," which creates the same stomach because alcohol destroys the liver. If you happen to have excess weight in the midsection, a glass of wine or beer at night will just make things worse.

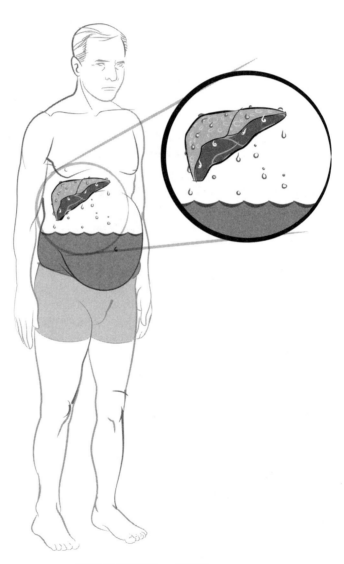

FLUID IN ABDOMEN—ASCITES

The pictures below show the changes from a normal body shape through the progressive stages of the Liver type.

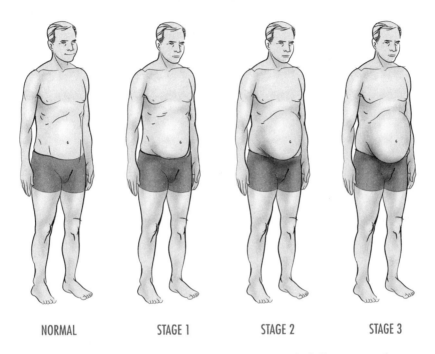

NORMAL   STAGE 1   STAGE 2   STAGE 3

Liver types usually have a dull pressure and fullness in the upper abdomen just under the right rib cage. Some of these people get tired for a while after each meal. When they lie on their left side at night, it becomes uncomfortable due to a swelling of the liver, which pushes into the diaphragm, cutting down the expansion of breathing. Lying on the right side seems to be the most comfortable. They are sensitive to a whole range of foods, especially fatty foods and refined grains, and must eliminate grains altogether or suffer the consequences of bloating, gas and indigestion.

There is a tight, almost arthritic-like feeling in the lower back, particularly in the morning. There is also a tightness or pain in the right shoulder or right side of the neck, which they will swear is an old injury, but treatments to the right shoulder never seem to resolve it long term. The reason is because the right shoulder is just the tip of the iceberg.

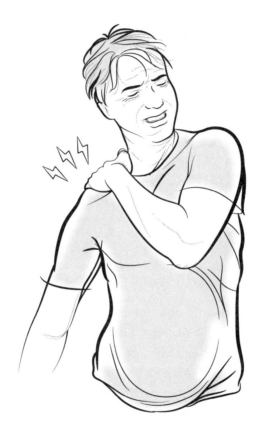

TIGHTNESS, PAIN AND STIFFNESS IN THE RIGHT SHOULDER OR NECK

The tongue has a deep split down the center and is often coated with a white film. The head frequently feels heavy and dull with aches in the forehead and neck area, and the person usually wakes up an hour before needing to get out of bed. In other words, the Liver type rarely gets the last part of sleep, resulting in inadequate sleep. The Adrenal type, on the other hand, sometimes gets up every 90 minutes or every two to three hours.

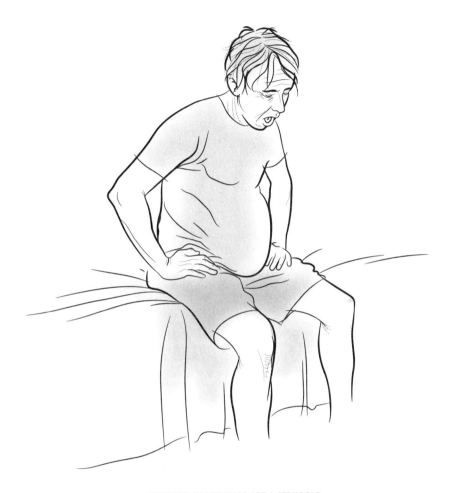

MORNING AWAKENINGS ARE A STRUGGLE

The morning is a struggle. This is because the liver can't hold blood sugar for a full seven hours; so morning grouchiness is actually coming from low blood sugar. When the person doesn't eat for a ten-hour span (from dinner to the next morning), the amount of sugar in the blood is excessively depressed, creating irritableness, moodiness, mentally depressed feelings and lethargy, most noticeable upon waking. Many Liver types become more pleasant to be around in the evening after several meals.

The urine is usually darker in the morning and becomes increasingly watery and clearer as the day progresses. Being similar to the oil filter in your car, the liver can get dirty.

The whites of the eyes can show a tint of yellow and can be very blood-shot in the morning as well. The eyelids may become itchy and swollen.

Arthritis and bad skin are also indicative of liver damage.[1] The finger joints, particularly in the morning, become stiff and slightly swollen. This worsens if refined grains were consumed the night before, since many Liver cases have difficulty with gluten (the protein part of grains). Wheat and other grain products seem to aggravate arthritis and cause joint pain and inflammation in various parts of the body (midback, low back, lower neck, hands, right shoulder, ankles and even in the knees).

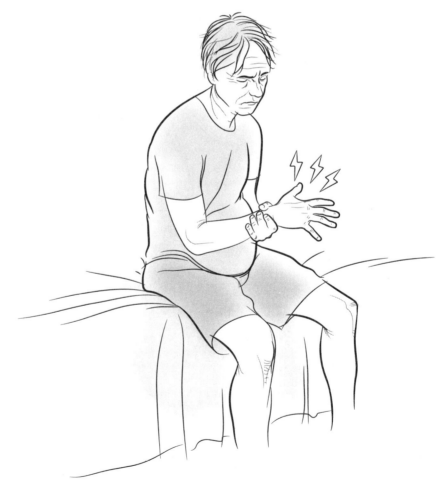

STIFF, SORE AND SWOLLEN FINGER JOINTS IN THE MORNING

When refined grains are avoided, the arthritis many times disappears. The body seems to misidentify the gluten in these grains as a microbe, creating an inappropriate immune response. The only grains that don't have gluten are rice, millet, spelt and oats. However, I'm recommending avoiding all grains on this diet.

Digestive problems are also a characteristic of the Liver type. This includes bloating, constipation and acid reflux.

Liver types will often crave the very foods that will destroy the liver — fatty foods, bacon, chips and deep-fried foods, especially from fast-food restaurants. When they are hungry, fried catfish, breaded onion rings or French fries look very appetizing. But after eating these foods, they will feel bloated, as their digestive systems are poor, and they'll usually start burping and belching after a high-fat meal.

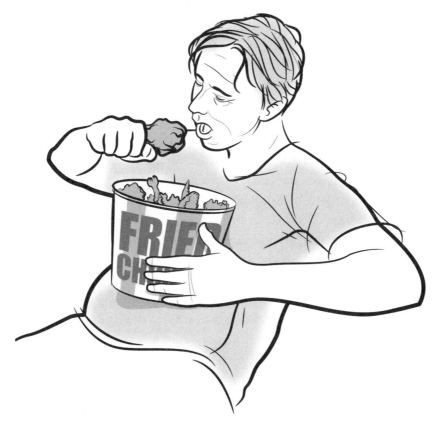

CRAVINGS FOR FATTY FOODS

If the liver is weakened, the person might get brown spots on the backs of their hands and throughout the body, called liver spots. Other skin issues that can occur are red dots, psoriasis, eczema, and even fungal growths on the scalp and toenails.

Itching is the most significant clinical symptom of severe liver cell damage.[2] The person seems to be always scratching something on their body; they experience itchiness especially at night. The itchiness usually occurs because the liver fluids are backing up into the blood.

With an advanced liver problem, the fingers occasionally look clubbed (blunted and squarish) and the nail beds appear whitened.[3] The nail bed should normally have a pinkish color.

As the liver becomes progressively more destroyed, the person's breath develops a distinct odor, musty and sweetish. If you ever visited a sick room in the hospital, you'd notice this smell.

Sometimes the bowel movements become light colored because of a lack of bile production. Bile is the substance produced by the liver that assists in breaking down fats. It's like the soap that dissolves the grease.

And because the liver has a main function of breaking down chemicals and environmental hormones, excessive estrogens can build up in the body. In major cases, a male body can start developing female characteristics—enlarged breasts, thinned skin and even a higher voice. Atrophy (shrinkage) of the testes can occur from this as well. Another side effect of excessive estrogens is spider veins. This is due to the blood vessel weakness caused by estrogens. As you might know, strokes are one of the negative side effects from hormone replacement therapy.

I have personally observed a loss of memory in many people with poor liver function. Even the medical textbooks describe "brain confusion" as part of liver problems.[4]

The liver can also be a source of high blood pressure and edema (swelling) in the ankles.[5] Blood needs to flow freely through the liver, so any obstructions within the liver (scar tissue) will create a back pressure.

Excessive scar tissue can occur in a damaged liver, a condition known as cirrhosis. In order to call it cirrhosis, however, it has to be major scarring; if it's only minor scarring it can't be called cirrhosis. It is my belief that many people have some minor scarring, enough to block liver function and cause weight gain and fluid retention in the abdomen. There are situations whereby cirrhosis is reversible, provided the damaging triggers are removed and sufficient time is allowed for a return to normal liver structure.

The liver is definitely one organ that has the capacity to totally rejuvenate. It is constantly repairing itself, yet there is a point where it gets overwhelmed.

Causes of the Liver Body Type

A liver problem can originate from many different sources. One is constipation. If the bowels cannot eliminate, the liver will become backed up. The toxicity in the body will prevent weight loss. A woman with this situation came to see me, who had received one of the introductory offers in my e-mail health tips inviting her to come in for a free consultation. When she showed up at the office, she was close to 400 pounds. She told me she had driven from Michigan to my clinic in Virginia for one consultation to help her lose weight. Then I found out she was having only one bowel movement per month! And she was more interested in weight loss. I explained that her bowels had to be handled before she could even think about losing weight. I never saw her again — her bowel problem wasn't a concern.

Another source is the consumption of refined sugars, which include hidden sugars such as juice and alcohol. The liver is the first line in the chain of organs that deal with sugar. When you eat lots of sugar, the liver is forced to handle it.[6] This creates major stress on the liver.

Sugar (as in cake, candy and other sweets) breaks down so fast it shocks the liver, making it weaker. On the other hand, vegetables break down so slowly you'll never have to worry about overeating them; the nutrition level is so high in vegetables that your body just won't let you eat too many. But if you take carbohydrates in their refined form — white sugar, alcohol, breads or even fruit juices — it's easy to overeat, since nutrition is low and the body won't tell you when to stop. Vitamin and mineral levels in food signal the brain and tell it when it is satisfied. Refined foods are stripped of their nutrition. The fiber in vegetables turns off the hunger switch as well.

What many people don't fully understand is that sugar, breads, pasta, cereals, crackers, pancakes, waffles, juice and soda are equally hard on the liver. All will be converted to either fat or cholesterol. The mixture of sugars with fats — in the form of ice cream, barbecue ribs and breaded meats — adds stress to the liver too.

Consuming excessive quantities of proteins and fats also puts damaging stress on the liver cells.

The liver produces substances to break down fats, but when it is deficient, an overload of fatty foods aggravates the liver. This shows up as tightness around the chest (just below the ribs), pain or tightness in the right shoulder area, belching or burping, and bloating in the digestive system.

Cravings for fatty foods come from the body telling you it needs something. What? It needs the fat-soluble vitamins — A, D, E, K and certain B vitamins. If you listen to your body, it will explain what it needs. Sausage, meatloaf, bacon, overly cooked greasy roast beef, deep-fried onion rings, French fries, breaded meats, greasy barbecue ribs, all are hard on the liver and its associated gallbladder. Eating raw beets (grated over salad) or steamed beets (not canned) each day will make the Liver type feel very good. Beets thin the bile and are also great for constipation.

A further big cause of liver problems is toxic chemicals. This is another way in which estrogens from the environment, along with pesticides and insecticides like DDT, adversely affect the body. These substances become trapped in the liver and create altered function.

Viruses and fungi can destroy the liver, hepatitis being a common liver problem. When a person takes excessive antibiotics, he or she can end up with all sorts of fungi, unfriendly bacteria, yeast and Candida. Candida is a yeast-like fungus that is normally in balance with other friendly microbes; but an overgrowth of Candida, which spreads on the tongue and private parts, can occur after antibiotic use. If you have this situation, to replace the good bacteria consume more fermented foods: pickles, apple cider vinegar, sauerkraut and plain yogurt (low-fat). It is not true that people with yeast need to avoid friendly yeast foods — just the opposite.

High-cholesterol drugs have been known to weaken the liver. Since many side effects from medications affect the liver, the liver is a common weak link in a large percentage of the population.

Liver damage could be brought about through nutritional deficiencies, especially the B vitamins. I'm not recommending going out and taking some synthetic vitamins, as they can create other problems. I would recommend avoiding refined foods, which deplete B vitamins. Breads, pasta, cereals and flour products are usually enriched with B vitamins because during the refining process B vitamins are destroyed. However, just spraying some synthetic vitamins doesn't fix this problem. Consuming refined grain products and refined sugar depletes the body primarily of B vitamins and potassium. A very good source of the B vitamins is nutritional yeast from the health food store. One teaspoon per day would be very wise. Make sure you don't confuse this with brewer's yeast or baker's yeast; get the nutritional yeast.

And by the way, synthetic B vitamins are made from coal tar, not food. Always consume vitamins from food. The foods must be listed on the label. If you see 50 mg of B_1, 50 mg of B_6, etc., then you can be pretty sure they are synthetic. Food concentrates come in smaller and different quantities, such as 3.4 mg or 32.4 mg.

Consuming processed prepared foods high in MSG (monosodium glutamate) damages the liver. This is a way to take massive quantities of sodium without tasting the saltiness of it. The next day the hands get swollen and the ankles have edema lines when you take off your socks, not to mention that blood pressure increases.

Many people avoid salt or sodium if they have high blood pressure. Why not increase the opposing mineral, potassium? In this program, you will be consuming large quantities of potassium-rich foods. High-potassium, low-sodium foods would be all the leafy greens, kidney beans, avocados, honeydew melon and sea kelp.

Testing for Liver Damage

Liver damage often will not show up on blood tests; even significant damage may show normal findings on liver tests.[7] The liver is rugged and takes lots of abuse, so there can be considerable damage before any symptoms are present. I had one patient who was an alcoholic from age 14 through 42. He has been dry for ten years but it's amazing he's not dead.

The most accurate way to determine liver damage is through a biopsy; of course, that's a bit invasive. Ultrasound of the abdomen can tell if the person is carrying fluid (ascites), but other tests might not tell the full story. Normal liver enzymes are not a good indicator of the absence of liver damage. Many people have normal levels yet have advanced liver disease.

Creating a Healthy Liver

Because all fat-burning hormones create their effects through the liver, having a healthy liver is the most important first step in weight loss. Without a healthy liver, fat burning will be next to impossible.

The best foods for the liver are raw cruciferous vegetables and small amounts of lean proteins (raw nuts, fish, etc.). Since a damaged liver has difficulty breaking down proteins, raw proteins such as those found in sushi (eaten without the rice) and sashimi are healthy for the liver. The raw fish is loaded with enzymes and is less stressful because it is raw rather than cooked. Cooked fish is the next best thing, then chicken and lamb. Eggs are also good unless the gallbladder is sluggish.

Red meats tend to be a bit more stressful to digest than fish, but in small quantities they are fine. A large cooked piece of meat is very stressful on the liver. As far as red meat is concerned, it's much easier for the liver to digest a rare steak than a fully cooked one. However, don't ask for a "rare" burger at the McDonald's drive-up window. I'm talking about a high-quality steak. A small amount of red meat would be okay a few times per week; but when you add the bun to the hamburger, it creates more stress on the liver.

In college, I don't think I ate even one vegetable. I told myself, "I'll eat healthy when I graduate." Boy, was that smart! Shortly after graduating I started getting liver symptoms and it took a long time for me to recover. To this day I still don't enjoy vegetables, but they are mainstays of my diet because now I know better.

I have one patient from the Philippines who lost 42 pounds of water weight from his stomach within six weeks of doing my program. Depending on the size of the belly, it could take two to six months to completely flatten the stomach; fat comes off gradually, while fluid weight can come off rapidly. Some people have to stay on the Liver Enhancement Plan for the entire time. But the potbelly comes off to the degree that you create a healthy liver. You can't take a person who has a lifetime of poor eating and expect two weeks of healthy eating to fix the liver. Unless you've been eating organic foods, the chances are good that you have been ingesting foods exposed to pesticides, insecticides, antibiotics, herbicides, fungicides and estrogen.

If a person has liver damage, cholesterol accumulation will usually occur, primarily because the liver is the main organ that breaks it down.[8] Lots of my patients with high cholesterol and even high blood pressure see excellent results from the Liver Enhancement Plan. In fact, this plan is beneficial for anyone who has high cholesterol.

Here's one success story that was sent to the person's medical doctor:

> "It is this program that enabled me to lower my cholesterol from 226 in May 2005 to 197 in March of this year. My triglycerides also dropped from 104 to 64 during this same testing period. Similarly, my wife's cholesterol dropped from 248 in June 2005 to 187 in March of this year. Basically our carbs come from fresh dark green vegetables. We are eating at least 4 ounces of animal protein with every meal, including eggs and hormone-free meats (chicken, fish, pork and beef). We eat virtually no grains, bread or pasta and have very little processed sugar intake. Additionally, I have lost 20 pounds since I started with the regimen."
>
> —RR, Centerville, VA

Cholesterol and Eggs

Since we are on the topic of cholesterol, you should know about the antidote (remedy) to cholesterol—lecithin. Rather than only avoiding cholesterol foods, it would be better to make sure you include foods high in lecithin. And you might be surprised that a very excellent source of lecithin is the egg yolk—the exact thing people who have high cholesterol are told to avoid. Even the derivation of *lecithin,* the Greek word *lekithos,* means "yolk of an egg." Eating eggs with yolks is beneficial for the liver, not only because of the high lecithin, but because they are a complete balanced food and easy to digest. However, if you have a sluggish gallbladder, fish would be a better source of protein. Gallbladder symptoms give you right shoulder pain, fullness in the right lower abdomen area and burping and belching after you eat. Personally, I eat a 4-ounce piece of fish for breakfast—it might sound strange, but my body runs better on that than other proteins. Twice a week I will have eggs.

Atherosclerosis

While on the subject of cholesterol, let me tell you my theory on what causes atherosclerosis (so-called clogged arteries). People have this idea that when they eat excessive fatty foods the cholesterol floats around in their arteries and starts to plug them up. This is not what happens. The plaque occurs not on the inside of the artery but within the inner lining of the artery. So it must be more an internal problem than cholesterol floating and plugging. Some other credible authors believe that what initiates this is a breakdown within the artery wall.[9]

The arteries are made of collagen, which is a protein. Therefore, hormones that destroy proteins must be involved in the process (excess cortisol and deficiency of growth hormone). This could be the reason people with adrenal problems bruise easily. Repair and maintenance of these arteries also require vitamin C. That is why people with vitamin C deficiencies get weaknesses within the blood vessels, as in bleeding gums, spider veins and varicose veins. Vitamin C helps in the formation of the collagen, or cement, that holds everything together. Vitamin E is the other vitamin that assists in the repair of tissues—it is the healing vitamin. I personally believe that in a vitamin C and E deficient state the person is very susceptible to atherosclerosis. Mushrooms provide an excellent source of vitamin C. Raw wheat germ is an excellent source of vitamin E; however, you don't need much— one teaspoon three times per week. Leafy green vegetables are the foods that contain both these vitamins.

Liver Spots

This leads to another topic—liver or aging spots, usually on the backs of the hands. There are many theories about this. My theory is that a vitamin E deficiency has something to do with creating this brown pigment. It could also come from the destruction of certain liver cells that make the pigment. Another cause could be a deficiency in a hormone from the pituitary gland in the brain that triggers the color of the skin.

What's interesting about this is that a good portion of the body's vitamin E is stored in the pituitary gland. That is because it is needed for making hormones, especially all the sex hormones in the ovaries— estrogen, testosterone, etc. During menopause when the ovaries shut down, a woman's vitamin E levels dramatically decrease due to the altered pituitary-ovary connection; and when the liver loses its vitamin E supply, a brown pigment gets released. I would recommend all women over the age of 50 consume a half-teaspoon of raw wheat germ every day to keep their vitamin E at a normal level. Wheat germ oil also works.

Growth Hormone

Growth hormone (GH) is directly associated with the liver and works through the liver. It is fat-burning and antiaging; it also controls the rebuilding of joints. A bad liver can prevent growth hormone from being produced. This shows up in excess fat, less lean body mass and squeaky joints (to put it technically).

I'm sure you have heard the hype on how GH is the fountain of youth. Growth hormone makes children's bones grow, regulates the size of your organs, decreases fat (fat burning), increases lean body mass, and controls sleep cycles the first half of the night. It rebuilds body tissue: joints, bone and muscle. Other hormones break down these proteins—for instance, the adrenal stress hormone cortisol.

Cortisol, if in excess, will eat up your thigh muscles, making it difficult to climb stairs or get up from a chair. In many cases, it's not growth hormone that is the problem but the cortisol that inhibits it. Years of stress, lack of sleep, bad foods, low-calorie diets, hard-core exercise, pain, inflammation and overactive adrenal glands can block growth hormone.

Many people take growth hormone without ever first finding out why they might be deficient—a poor liver. Growth hormone is made to protect, spare or save muscle, bone and joint proteins from being destroyed while at the same time keeping the fuel adequate between meals. The pancreas hormone insulin regulates fuel when you eat. Growth hormone regulates fuel between meals.

Since growth hormone is stimulated when you are not eating, we recommend, if you are a Liver type, not snacking between meals. Only consume three meals per day. The one exception is during the Liver Enhancement Plan, which will be covered in chapter 10.

Another activity that helps GH is exercise—not just any old exercise but intense exercise. There seems to be a direct relationship between growth hormone and the intensity of exercise, especially weight training and short, quick, intense types of sports. The problem is that cortisol is stimulated by stress and cortisol inhibits growth hormone. The trick is to trigger growth hormone without triggering cortisol. This means you need to do high-intensity, short-duration exercise with lots of rest in between. You'll learn more about this in chapter 14. Getting enough sleep also triggers growth hormone and for this reason fat burning occurs during sleep.

We've discussed what increases GH. Now let me mention what you need to avoid in order to prevent a decrease in GH. Sugar blocks GH. It's not sugar directly but the hormone that is triggered by sugar—insulin. Insulin is the fat-making hormone. Insulin changes carbohydrates (sugar) into fat and cholesterol. When insulin rises, growth hormone is blocked. This is why a belly full of carbohydrates before bed will inhibit GH from working through the night.[10] Even a small glass of juice or wine will prevent growth hormone through the night. I'm sorry, but that's the way it is.

Don't eat carbs at least 90 minutes before bed, especially the sweet ones. This includes hidden carbs such as beer, flavored yogurt and breads. You'd be shocked to find out what food manufacturers put sugar in these days— start reading labels and you'll see. You would burn more fat if you didn't eat anything before bed. I'm not saying never, but the more you stick to this, the more quickly fat will be burned. If you're going to drink, drink your alcohol in the morning (just kidding). Consuming carbs like juice, sugary sports drinks or so-called protein bars one hour before you work out can block growth hormone as well. I wouldn't even recommend eating fruit before working out.

Some of us just don't have time to sleep. I've had patients who get only three to four hours routinely. Getting less than seven hours per night can inhibit fat-burning hormones. If you are having sleep problems, there are several things you can do. Long walks during the daylight, reading a book before bed instead of watching TV, taking a calcium supplement (calcium with magnesium citrate), doing physical work around the yard, especially if you sit behind a computer screen, and consuming four celery sticks before bed are all good remedies.

Some research has found initial benefits from taking growth hormone: subjects on GH lost an average of 14.4 percent body fat and gained 8.8 percent lean body mass without diet or exercise.[11] The problem was that after several months of being on growth hormone, major side effects began: carpal tunnel syndrome, fluid retention, high blood pressure, joint pain, high blood sugar, diabetes, cancer, and inflammation in the pancreas.[12] This is because when you bypass your body's own production of GH, your body's production starts to decrease. Go ahead and take it if you have eight months to live. Other than that, I wouldn't recommend it.

Key Indicators

Key Liver type indicators are potbelly, brown spots on the backs of hands, yellowness in the whites of eyes, and poor joints. (See diagram on the next page.)

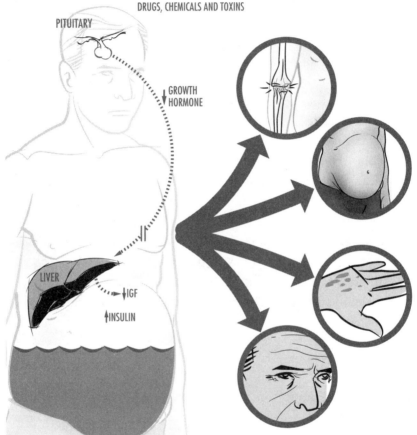

LIVER DESTROYERS

COOKED PROTEINS AND FATS

ALCOHOL

VIRUSES

ARTIFICIAL FATS

DRUGS, CHEMICALS AND TOXINS

ENVIRONMENTAL ESTROGENS

GROWTH HORMONES IN ANIMAL PRODUCTS

STEROIDS

REFINED SUGARS AND GRAINS

PITUITARY

GROWTH HORMONE

LIVER

IGF

INSULIN

COMMON LIVER ISSUES

IGF: Insulin-like growth factor. For more information on this hormone, see chapter 3, page 32, under "Fat-Burning Hormones," and chapter 9, page 125, under "Trigger #3."

Below is a list of symptoms the Liver type can experience from a poorly working liver.

Liver Type Symptoms

- Potbelly (very little external fat, mostly fluid)
- Brown spots on backs of hands and throughout body
- Poor joints
- Yellowness in whites of eyes (severe cases)
- Bloodshot eyes in the morning
- Eyelids itchy and swollen
- Hives and itchiness
- Skin problems
- Little red dots on skin
- Bloating after eating
- Burping or belching after eating
- Acid reflux
- Constipation
- Hemorrhoids
- Decreased tolerance for fatty foods and refined grains
- Cravings for fried foods and sour foods
- Chemical sensitivities
- Stiffness in lower back and upper back between the shoulder blades
- Pain or tightness in right shoulder area
- Liver roll of fat (just below the rib cage), seen mostly in women
- Dull pressure and sensation of fullness just under right rib cage
- Gallbladder problems
- Headaches
- Arthritis
- High cholesterol
- High blood pressure
- Varicose veins
- Spider veins
- Bad breath
- Tongue coated with white film

- Deep split down center of tongue
- Early morning insomnia (wake up one to two hours before alarm)
- Irritability and moodiness, especially in the morning
- Foggy brain in the morning
- Finger joints stiff, sore and swollen in the morning
- Fingers clubbed, with whitened nail beds
- Urine darker in morning, getting clearer during day
- Light-colored bowel movements
- Swelling in ankles
- Overheating of body, especially hot feet at night (not hot flashes)

9

The 10 Fat-Burning Triggers and Blockers

There are two basic types of problems with weight that need to be addressed: (1) fat and (2) water weight.

The first, actual fat, is a problem of a failing endocrine system (glands and hormones).

The second, fluid retention, is a problem of sodium and potassium imbalance, which could also be failing endocrine glands — adrenals.

Fixing both of these problems requires avoiding what has created them in the first place. Then actions need to be taken to restore glandular health. It's not just a matter of triggering your fat-burning hormones but, more importantly, avoiding those things that prevent fat burning and proper mineral balance. If you trigger fat-burning hormones without keeping the fat-making hormones to a minimum, you won't lose any weight, since all fat burners are nullified in the presence of fat-making hormones.

There are many ways you can attempt to lose weight. The high-protein, low-carbohydrate diets will help lower insulin but fail to balance sodium and potassium ratios. Potassium is needed to support fat-burning hormones. Low-calorie diets, on the other hand, will help temporary weight loss but will activate adrenal stress hormones, causing a rebound with a slower metabolism and more weight down the road. Low-fat diets can starve the body of raw materials for building fat-burning hormones, as these are made out of fat. High-fat diets can aggravate the liver, which is needed for all the six fat-burning hormones to work. High vegetable and fruit diets help with proper sodium and potassium ratios but fail to give enough protein to stimulate fat burning. The moderation diet of vegetables, so-called healthy whole grains and proteins is also not workable as far as hormones are concerned because "eating everything in moderation" (whole-grain foods, juice, wine or sugar) can block fat burning very easily.

In this program we will be smarter, by taking as many actions as possible to support hormone health while avoiding things that destroy hormone function.

Below are the ten very important factors in achieving this goal.

Trigger #1

The Absence of Sugar

Of all the things that have an impact on your metabolism, the most important one is sugar. Sugar triggers the powerful fat-making, fat-storing hormone insulin. In fact, in the presence of insulin not only will fat be blocked from being used as fuel BUT sugar will be converted to fat.

Sugar is a carbohydrate. And the most powerful trigger to fat burning is "the absence of sugar."

If given the choice of what it likes as a fuel source, the body will ALWAYS choose sugar as a preferred fuel over fat.[1] *This means that in order to burn fat, you can't have any sugar in the diet.*

Hidden sugars include vanilla yogurt or flavored yogurt, gum, alcohol, wine, beer, juice (especially orange juice), sports drinks, sodas, salad dressing with sugar, desserts, and even ketchup with high-fructose corn syrup. Many people have no idea of the number of hidden sugars in their diets.

Some people will try to convince you that chocolate and wine have powerful health benefits as antioxidants. Yet the amount of damage to your glands far outweighs any benefits from these antioxidants.

Other hidden sugars include **refined grains**, such as cereal, pasta, breads, crackers, pretzels, muffins, cakes, cookies, pancakes, waffles, donuts, rice cakes and puffed-rice cereals.

People have a big confusion about grains, which is contributed to greatly by promotion from the food industry: *Consume healthy whole-wheat grains instead of refined grains.* It doesn't matter if it's whole wheat or white bread; these starches turn into sugar fairly rapidly. Many people are also allergic to them, which leads to water retention and digestive troubles. I have found that cutting out grains is a very important factor in getting someone into fat burning. The only acceptable grain product in small amounts would be bran (the outer shell of the grain), which is high in fiber. Vegetable fiber is better quality because it has more nutrition, but fiber in general does slow the insulin hormone response.

Vegetable starches are also converted to fat. These would include potatoes, yams, corn, potato chips, French fries, hash browns, corn chips, etc.

Fruits, melons and berries have a higher sugar content than vegetable carbohydrates and can trigger small amounts of insulin; however, the fiber they contain acts as a buffer, slowing this response. **Bananas, dates, figs, raisins, canned fruit, dried fruits and mangoes** also have a high sugar content but with lower fiber and these have a greater effect on insulin. Some of the less sweet fruits are okay to eat on the Liver Enhancement Plan, as they tend to help eliminate water weight due to their high potassium levels. Apples are high in fiber and are definitely good to eat; in fact, I encourage a person to eat as many apples as he or she can throughout the day.

When you eliminate **sugary foods** like ice cream, candy, chocolate, added sugar to coffee and tea, and canned fruit with syrup, your body can tap into fat burning, because the trigger for fat release is *the absence of sugar.*[2]

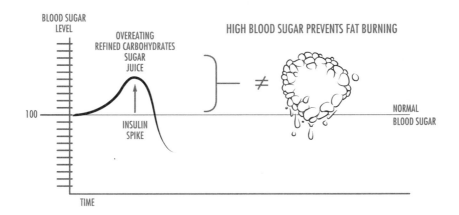

All aspects of fat burning are enhanced by the absence of sugar.[3] Cut out sugar as well as those foods that turn quickly into sugar and you'll automatically trigger fat-burning hormones. The best sugar substitute is the herb stevia (I recommend clear stevia). The next best sweeteners are either agave nectar, raw honey or Tupelo honey from the health food store—but use only if absolutely needed.

When sugar is not consumed, another hormone is triggered called glucagon. Glucagon does the opposite of insulin.[4] If insulin makes you fat, glucagon makes you thin. Glucagon is also triggered by protein (an adequate amount) and exercise.

The body has only a very small capacity to store sugar; anything over that will be automatically converted and stored as fat and cholesterol. To store sugar, potassium is needed. Without potassium, sugar storage is greatly limited and fat storing is enhanced. Sugar cane normally has lots of potassium, but when it's refined, potassium is lost. Therefore, if a person consumes refined white sugar, which is void of potassium, the body will store less sugar and make more fat and cholesterol.

Let me further clarify this by stating it another way: When the diet is deficient in potassium, the body is forced to store more fat than sugar; whereas when there is adequate dietary potassium, the body will store the sugar and convert less of it to fat.

Refined sugar also triggers sodium and water retention by decreasing potassium (opposing mineral).

Potassium is a body relaxer and calms the pulse rate. Since eating refined sugar depletes potassium, this increases the pulse rate, which you might have experienced as a pulsating pounding in the ears when you were trying to sleep.

If there is even a little bit of sugar in the diet, or if insulin is kept just slightly too high, fat fuel cannot be made available for energy. You could have the best diet throughout the day and then eat a small piece of something sweet at night and nullify all the good eating. With bad eating habits a person is constantly playing catch-up by working out twice as hard tomorrow or saying, "I'll eat better the next day to make up the damage from today."

Sugar will additionally block the fat-burning effects of exercise. For example, drinking a small amount of juice prior to exercising blocks the fat-burning hormones (especially growth hormone).[5]

In order for the diet to be successful, sugar needs to be completely eliminated. Once your body is healthy and you reach your ideal weight, then it will be able to tolerate occasional sugars, but not until you achieve your goal. Even drinking wine at night can set your liver back a few days.

Many people might not realize that the fat on their bodies actually comes from the sugar they eat, not from the fat they eat.

The same is true of cholesterol. Many people have high cholesterol not because they are consuming a lot of bacon or heavy fats but because they are eating large quantities of refined grains, sugars and starches.

This is a result of the influence of hormones over foods.

The graph below is an illustration to help you understand how the body responds to carbohydrates. Refined grains raise blood sugar, which spikes insulin and makes fat. Whole apples and whole carrots with fiber have little effect on insulin. The fiber buffers the insulin response. But when you refine them and juice them, blood sugars are elevated.

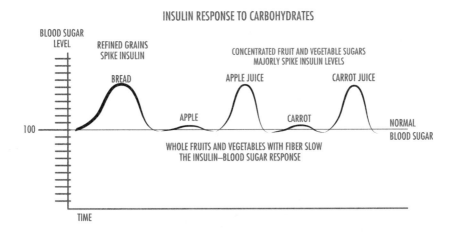

Excess sugar mixed with excess protein greatly increases insulin (fat-making hormone).[6] A sugary dessert after a large steak will increase insulin in a big way. Some other examples of this are BBQ Buffalo wings that contain sugar, breaded meats, meatloaf, ham, some deli meats that contain dextrose, or meat and potatoes. Protein without sugar only triggers insulin slightly; however, protein in general activates two other fat burners — glucagon and growth hormone.[7]

Insulin is the principal hormone triggered by refined carbohydrates and sugar. It is also a key hormone that stores fat. In the presence of any insulin, ALL other fat-burning hormones are nullified and blocked. So, not only is fat burning suppressed but fat is produced.

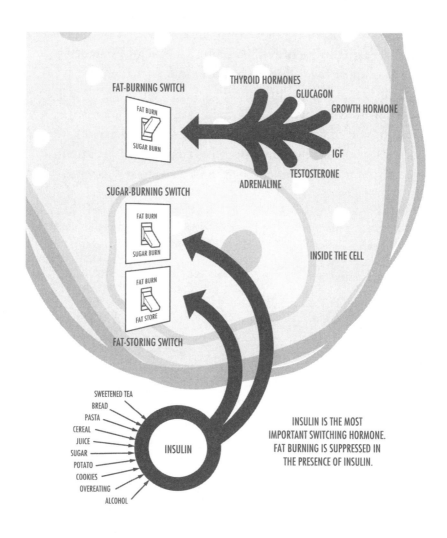

Trigger #2

Vegetables

Vegetable: *n.* of the plant family compared to the animal family. [Latin *vegetare*, "to enliven" < *vegetus*, "lively" < *vegere*, "to quicken," "wake." Late Latin *vegetabilis*, "animating"]

There are several important reasons why I included vegetables (non-starchy) in these triggers.

If the cause of your weight problem is a sick or failing endocrine system, then we need some nutrient-dense live food to heal it. The vegetable family has several qualities that aid in healing. Eaten raw, vegetables are one of the most concentrated sources of vitamins, minerals and plant chemicals. They are high in fiber, which buffers the fat maker insulin.[8] They are also low in sugar, even though they are called a carbohydrate.

Heat destroys nutrients. If the goal is to heal your body, then the more raw vegetables you eat, the faster this process will occur. Cooked vegetables will take away from the healing process. If you steam your vegetables, make sure they are lightly steamed, and also eat raw vegetables during the day. Ideally, you would consume 80 percent raw vegetables.

Vegetables have excellent ratios of high potassium and very low sodium. On the following page is a short list of high-potassium foods in milligrams. If you look at this chart, you can see that vegetables in general have very little sodium and high amounts of potassium. However, there are some vegetables that have high levels of sodium as well as high levels of potassium, such as beets and celery. These vegetables are beneficial for people with calcium deposits in their bodies, like gallstones and kidney stones, as sodium helps to balance the excess calcium.

The majority of overweight people are severely dehydrated in their cells and waterlogged outside their cells *despite* drinking lots of water. It sometimes takes up to six months of eating lots of vegetables to replace the potassium within the cells. You have to get it from food; taking a potassium supplement can't correct this problem. Processed, refined, boxed and canned foods do just the reverse: they create fluid retention because of the high sodium and low potassium.

Food	Amount	Potassium (mg)	Sodium (mg)
Apple	1 medium	158.70	0.00
Asparagus	1 cup	288.00	19.80
Avocado	1 cup	874.54	14.60
Banana	1 medium	467.28	1.18
Beef	4 oz	475.15	71.44
Beet	1 cup	518.50	484.50
Blackstrap Molasses	2 tsp	340.57	7.52
Broccoli	1 cup	505.44	42.12
Brussels Sprouts	1 cup	494.52	32.76
Cabbage	1 cup	145.50	12.00
Cantaloupe	1 cup	494.40	14.40
Carrot	1 cup	394.06	42.70
Cauliflower	1 cup	176.08	18.60
Celery	1 cup	344.40	103.40
Cranberries	½ cup	33.73	0.47
Grapefruit	½	158.67	0.00
Honey	1 oz	22.04	1.70
Kale	1 cup	296.40	29.90
Kidney Beans	1 cup	713.31	3.54
Lemon/Lime	¼ cup	75.64	0.61
Milk	1 cup	376.74	121.76
Mushrooms (crimini)	1 cup	635.04	8.51
Potato (with skin)	1 cup	509.96	9.76
Romaine Lettuce	1 cup	324.80	8.96
Rye	1 cup	148.72	3.38
Salmon	4 oz	572.67	68.04
Tomato	1 cup	399.60	16.20
Walnuts	¼ cup	110.25	0.50
Watermelon	1 cup	176.32	3.04

The nutrient profiles provided in the above chart are derived from
Food Processor for Windows, Version 7.60, by ESHA Research in Salem, Oregon, USA.

At my clinic we have a device that measures body fat and fluid levels, and the most startling breakthrough on this subject has been the discovery that many male patients coming into our office weighing between 250 and 350 pounds have normal or only slightly above normal body fat. However, they are full of fluid; and when someone has more fluid than fat, their sodium to potassium ratios are usually off. This is why the Liver Enhancement is best for them, as these foods are extremely high in potassium, which will slowly bring the water levels into a normal range. This works when you address the problem with whole foods. It doesn't work when you try to handle it with supplements. Any water weight problems always need high-potassium foods.

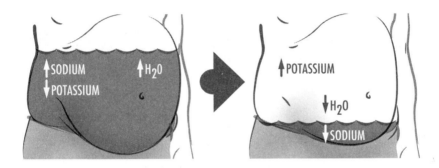

INCREASING POTASSIUM WILL DECREASE SODIUM AND WATER

Potassium helps lower insulin. Without enough potassium your insulin could increase and keep you out of fat burning. Potassium is also needed to adequately hold protein in your body (especially in the muscles). The electrical charge and energy of your cells are dependent upon incoming potassium. The best source of potassium, better than bananas, is vegetables.

Cruciferous Vegetables

Cruciferous vegetables have some very interesting properties; they are antiestrogen, anticancer, antitoxic chemical, and greatly help the liver in its ability to detoxify. Because estrogen is fat making and blocks the fat-burning growth hormone, eating many of these vegetables can help weight loss.

- Cabbage
- Brussels sprouts
- Broccoli
- Cauliflower
- Kale
- Radishes
- Turnips and turnip greens
- Bok choy
- Watercress
- Collards
- Mustard greens
- Rutabaga

Trigger #3

Protein

Protein is a powerful trigger for fat-burning hormones if it's not in excess. Protein stimulates two hormones — glucagon and growth hormone.

Now, there are two factors that should be discussed.

The first one involves the amount of protein. If you eat too much protein, insulin (fat-making hormone) can be triggered. Excess protein can create nearly the same insulin response as refined carbohydrates.

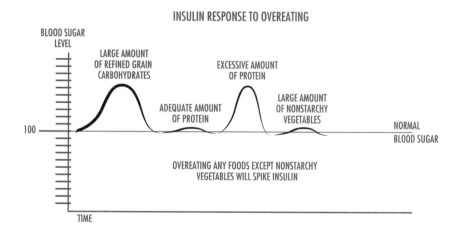

Your body can only absorb a maximum of 50 grams of protein at one sitting; this is about 7 ounces of steak. *But that is if you have a healthy liver. Most people with resistant weight have unhealthy livers and can't digest even close to that in one sitting.* So, with liver problems, eat less protein. If the thyroid is slow, the liver will not be able to process large amounts of protein. This is why I combine the liver and thyroid in one eating category.

The best thing is to eat smaller and more frequent protein meals — four to five times per day. However, if a person is mainly a Liver type, it's recommended they consume only three meals per day with no snacking in between, except while on the Liver Enhancement. This is because the liver's hormone, IGF, is stimulated between meals when the stomach is empty.

> IGF stands for insulin-like growth factor, which is a hormone the liver produces to regulate blood sugars between meals by releasing stored fuel (such as fat). It works in a similar way to growth hormone and is even triggered by GH.

If the liver is damaged and this hormone can't work, the pancreas is forced to pump out more insulin, which could lead to diabetes. So insulin and IGF work in tandem, insulin regulating the blood sugars during meals and IGF regulating blood sugars between meals.

You will be starting out with minimal amounts of protein, especially during the Liver Enhancement Plan, then increasing it as needed (if your body craves protein). The more damaged the liver, the less protein it can process. Eating high quantities of protein does not allow the liver to heal; that is why the Liver Enhancement Plan is vital to start the process. The liver is also responsible for removing waste from the consumption of protein.[9]

The key is to consume an adequate amount. Based on my own clinical experience, protein amounts depend on the body type or weakness. For example, a Liver or Thyroid body type requires a lot less protein and can't tolerate large quantities. In Liver cases, the processing or breaking down of protein is inhibited by a damaged liver. The way to stress the liver is to give it lots of protein at one sitting. A Thyroid body type also has difficulty with large amounts of protein because of slow metabolism. The Thyroid case works very slowly and the breakdown of protein is also sluggish. With the Liver and Thyroid body types, I would recommend using around 25 grams of animal protein per day. There is more about this in the diet section of chapter 11.

On the other hand, Adrenal and Ovary body types normally require additional protein (50–75 grams per day). An adrenal weakness can be very destructive in the breakdown of body proteins (muscles). This needs to be compensated for by adding more protein than is being broken down. The Ovary body type comes from an overabundance of estrogen, which makes fat. Increasing protein in the diet can trigger fat-burning hormones (like growth hormone) to counter the excess estrogen. You'll find more on this also in the diet section of chapter 11.

The second important factor with protein is consuming it in its whole form. Just as there are refined carbohydrates, there are also refined proteins. These would include protein powders and protein bars. Instead, consume whole eggs, raw nuts and seeds, cottage cheese, meat, fish, chicken, etc.

Consuming overly cooked protein can also be hard on the glands. This would include overdone beef, sausage, hot dogs, roasted nuts, milk (pasteurized) and peanut butter. If you eat peanut butter, eat some raw nuts during the day. In other words, if you eat cooked protein, balance it out with some raw protein. Raw proteins would be raw nuts, raw seeds, tahini butter, rare steak, sashimi or sushi (without the rice), and eggs that are runny. Yogurt and cheese are fermented and/or cultured and are considered partially raw; they have live enzymes. Of course, you wouldn't eat raw chicken meat. Hard-boiled eggs are okay to eat anytime.

Amino acids are the building blocks of protein. The amino acids arginine, glycine, tryptophan and valine are powerful stimulators of fat-burning hormones.[10] Instead of taking these in supplement form, why not get them from foods? You will notice that the recommended foods in this program contain highly concentrated fat-burning amino acids. These amino acids are present in cottage cheese, skim-milk yogurt, avocado, coconut, pecans, cashews, walnuts, almonds, Brazil nuts, hazelnuts, peanuts, pine nuts, pumpkin seeds, sesame seeds, sunflower seeds, beef, poultry (chicken and turkey light meat), wild game (pheasant, quail), seafood (halibut, lobster, salmon, shrimp, snails, tuna in water), eggs, chickpeas, winter squash, mushrooms, blueberries, grapes and oranges.

Protein can increase the fat on your body, but realize that nearly all of your body is made from protein and some of it needs to be replaced.[11] However, through initially decreasing protein and letting the liver heal, the body will become a lot more efficient at using protein through the help of growth hormone.

For the first two weeks of the Liver Enhancement Plan you will be eating pretty much all vegetarian foods. You will consume vegetarian proteins. After that, depending on your results, you might add some animal protein. I recommend animal proteins because they are more complete.[12]

One last point regarding animal proteins has to do with their quality. Consume organic (without hormones), grass-fed and wild-caught rather than commercial, grain-fed and farm-raised. The cancer-protective properties of healthy omega fatty acid ratios are much better, and for the body to heal, omega fats are necessary in their correct ratios. (Fatty acids will be discussed in more detail under "Essential Fats" in Trigger #4.)

In our program, we will start you out with very low proteins and gradually increase them until the correct amount for your body is reached. We have found this is the best approach for most people, due to the great imbalance of sodium and potassium. By initially feeding the person lots of high-potassium foods (vegetables) through the Liver Enhancement Plan, faster results can occur. This is because of a better sodium-to-potassium cellular ratio. And since excess animal protein can add more stress to the liver, cutting this out for two weeks makes increased liver function possible.

Trigger #4

Fats

Fats typically do not influence fat-making hormones; however, they do have the ability to stress the liver, which indirectly affects hormone flows through the liver.

The whole myth that fat is the big culprit making everyone fat doesn't pan out when you're talking about hormones. Fat has little effect on fat-storing hormones. Many people put too much importance on restricting fats in the diet. Yes, it is true that with Liver types low fats are best; however, this is not because fat turns into fat, but because fat stresses the liver.

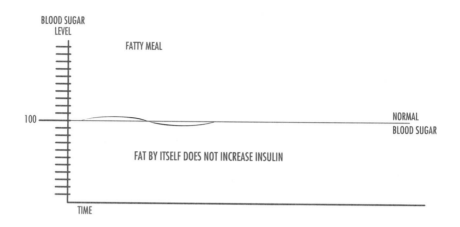

The benefits of a low-fat diet have even been rejected in the mainstream media as a factor in lowering risk for disease. And we wonder why people are so confused about nutritional facts.

There are also studies showing that a low-fat diet inhibits the fatburning hormone testosterone. This is why you need to include nuts, seeds, avocados, flax oil and olive oil in your diet, as well as the other fats listed in this section.

What most people don't understand is that carbohydrates (breads, sugars, wine, juice, etc.) are changed into fat and cholesterol much more readily than fat and cholesterol foods are turned into adipose tissue and increased blood cholesterol. In other words, low-fat cookies will make fat and cholesterol faster than cholesterol-laden eggs will. And eggs are rich in the antidote to cholesterol—lecithin.

An important point to know about cholesterol is that when dietary intake of cholesterol foods is high, the body will make less, and when dietary cholesterol intake is low, the body will make more.[13] This explains why many people still have high cholesterol despite consuming less of it.

It is also often not understood that cholesterol is only present in animal products and is not found in nuts, avocados, seeds or olives.

Another interesting factor concerning fat and cholesterol is that a good portion of your body is made of fat—brain, nerves, hormones and glands. Your body is constantly replacing these tissues with dietary fats. So, despite fats having more calories per gram compared with carbohydrates, some of these fats are used to replace body parts. This is especially true under stress, as the adrenals need to build more stress hormones. Carbohydrates are not used to replace body parts but are used only for fuel and vitamin and mineral supply. This is why excess carbohydrates are readily converted to fat as storage.

Hormonally speaking, eating carbohydrates is much more devastating for weight gain than the consumption of fat; and some studies even show that you will lose more weight on a high-fat, low-carbohydrate diet than on a low-fat, high-carbohydrate diet.[14]

Satisfying Effect

Cravings come from letting your blood sugars drop too low. When you eat fats, hormones are triggered to make you feel satisfied and eliminate the cravings. Carbohydrates, on the other hand, will not trigger these hormones but will do the opposite and inhibit the satisfying effect, causing more hunger. This is why eating sugar and refined carbohydrates will create a desire to consume more an hour later. Many people are eating the wrong foods, which keeps them craving and hungry all the time. Eggs — especially with the yolks — raw nuts, avocados and cheese are excellent foods to stimulate certain hormones and to decrease hunger and cravings.[15]

If a person craves sweets after a meal, they are usually deficient in or missing in their diet the amino acid tryptophan. Taking 500 mg of L-tryptophan before bed will usually help these cravings fairly quickly. This amino acid turns into serotonin and is good for depression as well as sleep.

Essential Fats

Essential fats are fats that are vital to the body yet cannot be made by the body. These essential fatty acids, as they are called, MUST be received from your diet. They include what are called the omega 3 and omega 6 groups.

Not eating enough **omega 3** fats—for example, fish, fish oil, walnuts or flax—will create an imbalance with other fats. Flax oil is one of the best sources from which to get your omega 3 fats, and I recommend you consume this liberally.

Omega 3 fatty acids have been shown to help prevent cancer. Grass-fed beef, wild-caught fish and free-range chicken are all very high in omega 3 fats and contain far more omega 3 than their grain-fed, farm-raised and caged counterparts. Apparently there are studies that show that eating red meat causes cancer. I would like to see a study done on the consumption of grass-fed beef versus corn-fed beef. As the ratio of omega 3 in the former is so much higher, my guess is that you would see a significant reduction in cancer among the group eating the grass-fed meat.

Omega 6 foods include sunflower seeds, sesame seeds, pumpkin seeds, evening primrose oil, borage oil, olive oil and olives, almonds, pine nuts, pistachio nuts, Brazil nuts, walnuts, hazelnuts, peanut oil—unprocessed (hard to find)—and avocados. Many of these foods have a combination of both omega 3 and omega 6 fats. Even grass-fed beef and free-range chicken, as well as eggs from free-range chickens, have a combination of omega 3 and 6, and grass-fed meats in general have far greater quantities of omega fats than grain-fed animals.

You need a 1:1 ratio of omega 3 and omega 6 fats.

The requirement for these fats (in nut and seed form) should be at least one handful per day. Getting them directly from food is better than using a supplement; however, any form is better than none at all. These essential fats supply the raw material with which to make cell walls and are used as well in the structure of your mitochondria (cellular energy factories). If building a house needs wood, your cells need omega fats, and their presence in the body enables oxygen to travel easily through the cells. There are very credible studies showing that cancer grows in areas of your body where a decrease in oxygen occurs. Essential fatty acid deficiencies are behind this decreased oxygen situation and are also a prime cause of dry skin and hair.

Trans Fats

Also known as trans fatty acids and hydrogenated or partially hydrogenated fats, these are man-made or processed fats, produced by adding hydrogen gas to a liquid fat or oil to make it thicker or more solid. This increases its shelf life, as it is less likely to spoil.

If you are consuming trans fats (margarine, artificial butters, either partially or completely hydrogenated), your liver will be stressed. They are like edible plastic and are very hard on the liver. Acceptable fats to use in place of these are olive oil, flax oil, safflower oil, butter and coconut oil.

The best cooking oils are coconut oil, safflower oil, olive oil and peanut oil. I recommend that you cook with coconut oil, since it has been demonstrated to have a positive effect on metabolism. The other good point about coconut oil is that it doesn't require much of the liver's bile to break it down, which means less stress on the liver. Bile is the detergent that breaks down grease or fatty foods.

Saturated Fats

Saturated fats are found mainly in animal products and also in certain plant foods.

Consuming excessive heavy saturated fats, such as bacon, sausage and overcooked beef, can stress the liver and especially the gallbladder. If a person has a healthy liver, some better-quality saturated fats can help with weight loss. The fats I recommend are coconut oil, butter, avocado, cream, cream cheese, rare steak and hamburger.

Eating more fat can sometimes increase the burning of stored fat.[16] I have had patients finally lose weight when they started increasing fats in their diets—avocados, butter and coconut butter. When the body receives this fat, it activates more fat-dissolving enzymes (lipases—things that break down lipids, or fats); also, fat has the antidote to cholesterol—lecithin. If you restrict fats in the diet, the body compensates by slowing the breakdown of fats; it goes into a holding mode. I have found that when a person who is trying to lose weight and doing everything correctly is still having a hard time, adding more fat can sometimes speed up weight loss.

A rule of thumb is *the worse the liver, the less fat you can tolerate in your diet.* Consume low-fat cottage cheese, low-fat yogurt and go very light on the oils—this includes peanut butter. Some people cannot even tolerate too many raw nuts; however, one handful of seeds or nuts would be easily tolerated by most.

The Adrenal and Ovary body types require more fats than the Liver and

Thyroid types. In the initial program, you will start out with very low fats, then over time gradually increase them to your optimum level.

Trigger #5

Skipping Meals, Reducing Calories or Letting Yourself Get Hungry

When you skip meals or do a fasting program, your blood sugars decrease, stimulating several hormones. The stress hormone cortisol (from the adrenals) increases, which turns your body tissues (muscles from the legs, buttocks and arms) into sugar fuel.[17] This is a survival mechanism to provide quick energy or to help you stay alive during starvation. However, as you learned in chapter 5, if this sugar is not completely burned up, it will be changed into fat and specifically deposited around your vital organs in the abdomen.

Lowered blood sugar from skipping a meal also creates cravings for the wrong foods — sweets. These then cause an increase in blood sugar, signaling another hormone — insulin — to come in and remove it from the blood. Where does it go? It is again converted into fat around your belly.

The rule of thumb here is EAT BEFORE YOU GET HUNGRY and NEVER SKIP A MEAL, ESPECIALLY BREAKFAST. One action is to keep raw nuts (walnuts and almonds) available at work or in your car. Another is to keep cheese, apples or cut vegetables available so that you have something to eat between meals. Unless you have a Liver body type, I recommend you eat frequent meals (four to five smaller meals throughout the day). This keeps a constant fuel source and prevents unnecessary destructive hormones from being triggered. It will also prevent cravings for sweets several hours later. These actions will keep cortisol from putting fat on your stomach and prevent the breakdown of muscle tissue.

There seems to be a huge confusion about calories. Calories are units of energy in food. What is being taught broadly is that excess calories cause weight gain and decreased calories cause weight loss. Too many calories absolutely can trigger weight gain from the powerful fat-making hormone insulin. But cutting calories will also trigger fat-making hormones and make you fat.

Understanding the dynamic aspects of hormones can give you an advantage in losing weight. For example, when you eat a low-calorie, low-fat bran muffin, insulin is activated, which not only converts the muffin into fat but prevents any burning of stored fat. However, consuming fats, which have higher calories, doesn't have this same effect; in fact, fat doesn't trigger insulin. That is why a tiny piece of low-fat, low-calorie candy can actually prevent the loss of fat much more than a fatty piece of low-carbohydrate cheesecake.

Trigger #6

Gland Destroyers

Alcohol (beer, wine or mixed drinks)

Not only does alcohol trigger insulin and cause weight gain but it also destroys the liver. Just a little alcohol at night can set your liver back for several days. What I mean by setting the liver back is preventing the liver from burning fat. The positive fat-burning effects from foods and exercise can likewise be canceled out by alcohol. You can eat really well and then that small amount of alcohol at dinner can keep you out of fat burning. Alcohol can also trigger the destructive hormone cortisol, since alcohol puts stress on the body. This constant irritation causes inflammation and scarring of the liver, which, in some cases, will not show up on blood tests until it is in the advanced stages.[18] Major scar tissue in the liver is the condition known as cirrhosis. Some people can get away with drinking alcohol merely because their livers and endocrine glands have not yet been destroyed.

Caffeinated Products (coffee, soda, tea and chocolate)

Caffeine stimulates and weakens the adrenal glands and liver and also irritates the gallbladder. It increases cortisol, which can put fat into and around the abdominal organs. If the adrenals are in very bad shape, I don't recommend coming off caffeine too quickly, as lethargy and other withdrawal symptoms can last up to three days, though in most cases it's one to two days. I would recommend cutting down to one small cup of coffee in the morning and then gradually lessening the amount over a two-week period until it's eliminated altogether. It has been shown that drinking two and a half cups of coffee can more than double the stress hormone adrenaline.[19] Even though adrenaline is a fat-burning hormone, the increased cortisol counters this effect. Cortisol tends to stay in the bloodstream much longer — up to eight hours. A sick liver will not be able to rid itself of cortisol very well, causing this hormone to stay in the body even longer. Increasing cortisol lowers growth hormone (fat-burning and antiaging); and because cortisol is being released, excess stored sugar is being released, causing insulin to convert it to fat around the stomach.

The liver is forced to detoxify the caffeine from coffee; this puts more strain on the liver. I recommend switching to Roma (a coffee-like beverage) or organic water-processed decaf coffee, as commercial decaffeinated coffees can contain toxic chemicals used in removing the caffeine.

Appetite suppressants are stimulants, which in many cases have caffeine. They even sell caffeine in pill form at the gas station to help truck drivers stay awake. Herbal stimulants, which do not have caffeine, can have the ability to stimulate and burn out your glands — including ma huang (ephedra), guarana, gotu kola and kava.

Sodas, tea and chocolate also contain caffeine and so have the same effect. Caffeine, in addition, depletes calcium and B vitamins from the body. Other than that, it is totally fine! Sparkling water is a good substitute. Herb tea (decaffeinated) is likewise a good alternative. Green tea is another beneficial way to transition because, despite having some caffeine, it has an anticaffeine effect; but here again, naturally decaffeinated green tea would be the better choice.

Drugs

Recreational drugs and medications of all kinds have side effects on the glands, especially the liver. Psychiatric drugs deplete hormones and also make it hard to lose weight. Hormone-replacement hormones and birth control pills both contain estrogen, which is a fattening hormone. Prednisone is an anti-inflammatory steroid (adrenal hormone), which is also fattening. Insulin is a fat-making hormone. Anticholesterol and blood pressure medications have side effects on the liver as well. Diuretics deplete minerals, which can affect the adrenal glands. Antibiotics kill your friendly bacteria, putting stress on your liver because of stress on digestion. These chemicals and others can be big barriers to losing weight. However, I'm not suggesting you come off your medication without the advice of a competent medical doctor.

Detoxification (*toxin* meaning "poison," + *de-*, "to remove")

The liver is the main organ that is supposed to eliminate these chemicals, in two phases. In the first phase the liver tries to neutralize toxins. In the second phase it will try to convert the neutralized toxins into less harmful particles, which can be eliminated through the urine and bowel.

The following are examples of substances handled by the liver in phase I and II detoxification: drugs, steroids, heavy metals, fertilizers, solvents, environmental estrogens, food additives and dyes, sulfites added in salads you buy in the grocery store (salad bars), sulfites in wines, nitrates in deli meats, synthetic perfumes and makeup absorbed through the skin, alcohol, antibiotics, cigarette smoke, protein waste from high-protein diets, pesticides, exhaust fumes, charcoal-grilled meats, paint fumes, viruses, bacteria, yeast, Candida, fungus and molds. Your own excess hormones are also either deactivated or recycled within your liver.

There are specific foods that the liver needs in the process of detoxification. These foods include the cruciferous vegetable family: cabbage, broccoli, Brussels sprouts, kale, radish and collard greens. However, beets are especially important in phase II and help additionally with the deactivation of estrogens. I have found that patients who include half a beet in their diets each day (raw, grated on salads, or steamed, not canned) start noticing increased sex drive and improved lean muscle mass. I believe this is due to decreased estrogen, allowing testosterone to come to its normal level. Beets also allow for the clearing of the stress hormones cortisol and adrenaline, which is great for people who have anxiety, constipation or sleep problems.

Growth Hormones

The animals whose products we eat (meats, milk, cheese), including farm-raised fish, are fed growth hormones. Some are estrogens and some are a type of growth hormone. It is my personal opinion that these hormones have greatly damaged our endocrine glands. For more information on this, see "What Causes Gland and Liver Problems?" in chapter 3.

Endocrine Disruptors

As covered in chapter 3, pesticides, insecticides, heavy metals, etc., all can mimic estrogen within your glands. These chemicals are on the golf course, in the schools, in restaurants, in your garden, and on your vegetables unless you eat organic. Being exposed to DDT as children, or consuming fruits that have been sprayed with DDT and shipped in from third-world countries, has damaging effects on us. Vaccines also have heavy metals and formaldehyde in them. The amalgam (mercury) in our teeth and the mercury in tuna can affect our hormones. I would recommend switching to organic, hormone-free foods as much as possible (at least 50 percent).

Food and Cosmetic Chemicals

Food preservatives, food dyes, synthetic sugars (dextrose), hydrogenated oils, and even things like synthetic vanilla flavoring all have a bad effect on our glands. Also, skin creams, makeup, shampoos and perfumes can easily absorb through the skin and end up in your liver. Did you know if you rub some garlic or an onion onto the bottom of your foot that within 10 minutes you'll be able to taste garlic or onion? Creams, lotions and cosmetics do absorb through your skin and, through the bloodstream, travel to the liver. Your skin is an indicator of the health of your liver. It is ironic that people are trying to make their skin look better through cosmetics, when these are the very things that are worsening their skin.

Consuming Food without Enzymes

Enzymes are proteins that do ALL the work of the body. Without enzymes, body reactions would take years to occur. Enzymes not only help you digest but help rid your liver of toxic chemicals, stop inflammation, reduce blood pressure and cholesterol, regulate temperature, make hormones, and build body tissues such as hair, nails and skin. Enzymes are the workhorses of the body, and when you consume food without enzymes, you are depleting your enzyme reserve.

You could look at the body as an enzyme bank or reserve. Let's say you ate some food without the enzymes to break down fat (called lipases); your body would then have to release its own lipase reserve. Over time, you can exhaust this supply, creating strain on the glands and organs. Animals that were fed roasted nuts, for example, developed enlarged pancreases, since the pancreas is the key organ to produce and release enzymes. In other words, consuming cooked, steamed, pasteurized, roasted, processed or refined foods forces your body to deplete its enzyme bank, leaving you with degenerative disease.

The first area to repair in an enzyme-depleted body is the glands. This is why we start you out with lots of raw, enzyme-rich foods.

Trigger #7

Water Retainers

A huge hidden source of being overweight is water weight.

When people come into our clinic weighing 250 to 350 pounds with normal or just barely over the normal amounts of body fat, it startles them to realize that most of their weight is water weight.

For example, a 30-year-old male weighing in at 264 pounds had body fat of 24.6 percent. Normal body fat for his age and height is 24.6 percent. In other words, his body fat percentage was perfect, yet his belly was huge. I found out he was loading up his body with massive quantities of hidden fluid retainers. He couldn't believe it when I told him he was not fat.

Another 40-year-old patient weighing in at 350 pounds had 35.7 percent body fat. His normal should have been 26.5 percent. That's only 9.2 percent above normal — not bad. His doctor had told him previously to drink two and a half gallons of water per day to flush out his fat. I put him on the Liver Enhancement Plan and he's losing weight steadily every week and feeling great. He needs to be on the Liver Enhancement for six to eight months with some fish protein every day, as his body craves it.

Monosodium glutamate is the big culprit in causing water retention and it can be hidden under a variety of names: modified food starch, autolyzed yeast, calcium caseinate, sodium caseinate, hydrolyzed protein, hydrolyzed vegetable protein, carrageenan, glutamic acid and yeast extract. MSG is also present in most protein isolates (soy isolates, whey isolates, etc.). Many Chinese restaurants will tell you they don't add MSG, yet it's in their sauces under other names. I can taste if food has MSG — it tastes just a bit too good and I can keep eating more than usual; but the next day my finger joints ache and feel puffy.

Many boxed foods, canned foods, gravies, sauces, mixes, TV dinners, lunch foods, hot dogs and condiments have either MSG or lots of chemicals or preservatives that cause water retention. Eating at restaurants gives you a good dose of MSG. It's a difficult substance to avoid. When dining out, keep away from breaded foods and foods with creamy sauces. Eat whole foods with just a few spices. If it is unavoidable, counter the sodium with lots of leafy greens or vegetables, which are high in potassium.

When shopping, make sure you read the labels, especially for the sodium amounts, as you will find that most packaged and processed foods contain mega sodium. They don't list potassium unfortunately, which is the opposing mineral. I have found a product called Kettle Chips to have higher potassium than sodium. However, potato is a starch and will not help you lose weight.

An additional note on MSG: In animal studies, MSG has been shown to triple the output of insulin. Insulin is not only the major fat-making hormone, it is the main preventer of fat burning. In the presence of insulin, your body can NOT burn fat.

Artificial sweeteners, which are in thousands of foods, cause water retention, especially the diet sodas that so many people drink. These include aspartame, saccharin and acesulfame K. Sugar alcohols, such as

Splenda, xylitol or mannitol, are another type of artificial sweetener. I initially did recommend sugar alcohols as acceptable sweeteners but with more of my own research found that they are big water retainers, so I don't recommend them anymore.

Excess sodium causes increased water retention and decreases potassium. The adrenal hormones are affected indirectly when this mineral imbalance is created.

A major hidden source of potassium-depleting, sodium-retaining foods is refined sugars and carbohydrates. In order to digest sugar, potassium is required. And because potassium is not normally present in white sugar or white flour, you end up using your potassium reserves. Since the cell is where most of the potassium is located, a depletion of this mineral will cause dehydration in the cell with fluid retention outside the cell. This is why you feel puffy and have ankle swelling after eating something sweet, and why consuming sweets makes you thirsty. It is also why you can gain and lose five pounds in a day or gain five pounds overnight. It isn't fat; it's water, which comes with the increased sodium.

Alcohol causes water retention as well.

It would be a good idea to take a look at how many water retainers you are exposed to on a weekly basis and compare this to how many high-potassium foods you eat.

Trigger #8

Exercise

A very interesting yet rarely understood fact of exercise is that the calories burned during exercise are very few. For example, it would take 1 hour of golfing (walking without a cart) to burn several teaspoons of Thousand Island dressing. However, the delayed fat-burning effects from this exercise are quite significant. You experience most of the fat burning 14 to 48 hours after the exercise — BUT only if certain things are in place. Burning this fat depends on what you eat during this time, how much stress you experience, whether you have pain or not, how much you sleep, and if you are avoiding sugar completely. This is why you don't have to pay too much attention to calories, only to hormones; if you do this, you'll be much more successful.

Eating carbohydrates before, during or after you exercise will prevent the fat-burning effects.[20]

You have probably been told, "Eat everything in moderation," right? This is bad advice. Eating sugar even in small amounts will keep you out of fat burning. Eat protein at least 75 minutes before exercising—but don't stuff yourself. It is okay to eat protein after the exercise as well.[21]

Exercise inhibits the fat-making and fat-storing hormone insulin.[22]

Intense anaerobic (higher-pulse-rate or resistance-type) exercise triggers several fat-burning hormones—growth hormone, testosterone, adrenaline and glucagon.[23] However, if the adrenal glands are fatigued or exhausted, intense exercise can prevent weight loss because the stress glands are being overtaxed. If your adrenals are stressed, only do light aerobics (low-pulse-rate endurance-type), if any at all, until you get your energy back and your sleep is improved.

Anaerobic exercise: Higher-pulse-rate (greater than 145 beats per minute), intense resistance-type.

Aerobic exercise: Low-pulse-rate (less than 130 beats per minute) endurance-type.

It's true that the low-pulse-rate (aerobic) exercise burns fat during the time you are doing it, but only after the first 20 to 30 minutes. So if you exercise 40 minutes per day, this is only 10 minutes of fat burning—very insignificant. On the other hand, the intense, high-pulse-rate (anaerobic) exercise does not burn fat during the exercise, but triggers fat-burning hormones 14 to 48 hours later.

During the exercise, you are tearing down muscle tissue and causing cortisol to help break down muscle. Then the growth hormone comes in to repair and rebuild it. The fat-burning benefits occur in the rest period when the body is building back up. There is more on this in chapter 14, "Exercising for Your Body Type."

Trigger #9

Stress

Stress can severely affect your weight.

Stress increases the hormone cortisol, which can lead to fat being deposited in and around the abdomen.[24] This is because the adrenal hormone releases a good supply of stored sugar (from both liver and muscles) into the bloodstream, causing insulin to change it into fat.

Types of stress could be contact with poison ivy, receiving a burn or an injury, loss of a loved one, fighting with your spouse, dealing with an angry employer, constipation, not sleeping, getting a hot flash, watching the news (usually negative), reading the newspaper (death, scandal, hurricanes) or hanging out with negative people, as well as having pain or inflammation in your body. If you have pain, cortisol is raised. Pain can prevent weight loss because the hormone cortisol raises sugar and blocks fat from being burned. At present I am doing some in-house studies on the reduction of cortisol.

I have developed a stress-reducing procedure called Acupressure Stress Elimination Technique, which assists in getting rid of body stress, improving sleep and relieving tension. But it takes a trained practitioner to perform this procedure. To learn more and to locate a certified practitioner in your area, go to http://www.drbergacupressure.com/.

Exercise can reduce stress; however, exercise can also increase stress on the body because it increases cortisol. The goal is to exercise in a way so as to not raise cortisol too much. This would mean keeping your pulse rate low during exercise. Weight training is resistance-type exercise and increases cortisol unless you do fewer repetitions and rest between them. You also would not want to exercise over soreness.

A few antistress activities include walking, hiking, slow endurance-type exercise, being outside, working around the yard, avoiding the computer screen, and avoiding reading the newspaper or watching the five o'clock TV news station. Try reading a book before bed instead of watching TV.

Trigger #10

Sleep

The fat-burning growth hormone is active throughout the night while you sleep; however, it increases during the first two hours of deep sleep, especially between midnight and 4:00 a.m.[25] Omitting this sleep can prevent the fat-burning effect. In other words, the reason why you burn more fat during sleep is because the fat-burning growth hormone spikes during deep sleep cycles. It's difficult to catch up on that important sleep if you miss this time period.

CIRCADIAN RHYTHM AND GROWTH HORMONE

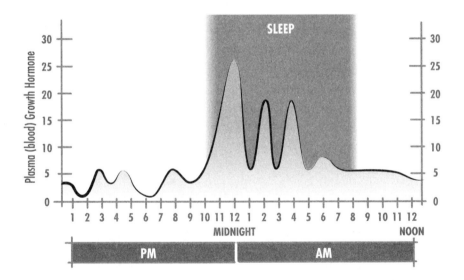

When you sleep, you typically go through four 90-minute cycles of light and deep sleep. Light sleep is REM (rapid eye movement) sleep, which is very active, producing lots of dreaming that you can remember. Delta-wave sleep is the deepest, in which you can dream but usually can't remember the dreams. Not getting quality sleep or getting inadequate sleep (less than seven hours) can prevent fat burning. You burn fat in the deeper sleep cycles, which could be a huge barrier for many people. You can't induce a deep rejuvenating sleep artificially through medication and expect to get these fat-burning effects; it has to be real natural sleep.

The delayed fat-burning effects of exercise can be prevented if you are not sleeping or if you eat sugar before, during or after exercise. If cortisol (stress hormone) is too high, not only will deep rejuvenating sleep be prevented[26]—which will affect the fat-burning growth hormone—but fat will be directed to and stored in the belly.

Eating before Bed

Eating or drinking refined sugars before going to bed (for example, orange juice) can nullify growth hormone's fat-burning effects as well as keep insulin high enough to prevent any fat release.[27] This includes a glass of wine. An apple, which has fiber, is a better snack before bed.

10

Step ONE: Liver Enhancement

Everyone should start with the Liver Enhancement, regardless of specific body type or mixed body type.

This Liver Enhancement eating plan will quickly get your body into fat burning. It is known that eating only protein and fat puts someone in ketosis (fat burning); however, I have found this eating plan has the same effect but without the stress on the liver that happens with high protein and fat diets. Purchase some ketone strips at the drugstore and check it out for yourself.

All six fat-burning hormones do their work through the liver. In fact, as we covered earlier, 80 percent of your thyroid function occurs through the liver.

Here's how the plan works:

You will be on this enhancement for at least 14 days.

The first 3 days might be a bit rough for certain people, as the body is switching from running on sugar fuel to running on fat fuel. But, surprisingly, most people actually feel very good on this part of the program. Your body's receptors for sugar have to be readjusted; after this program you'll find you will need less sugar, which will result in fewer cravings for sweets. Also, coming off caffeine can create some tiredness; this typically lasts for 1 to 2 days. The 4th day will be easier, and so on. Your energy usually starts to improve as your sleep becomes deeper. You'll find you are not as hungry, but do not skip meals. Other benefits noted are weight loss, inches lost, reduced aches and pains, improvement in skin and nails, and some people experience an increased sex drive. As the liver improves, fat can be made more available for energy.

On the 14th day of the program—depending on your results—you will either continue with the Liver Enhancement for a longer period of time or start adding some animal protein with each meal as you transition into the body-type diets. This is true whether you have a specific body type or a mixed body type. In other words, you won't automatically switch to the next diet at the end of the 14 days. In fact, if you are doing well and losing weight, are not craving protein or getting fatigued, I recommend you stay on the Liver Enhancement for as long as you can before going to the next step. This transition and how to judge when to start adding protein will be covered in more detail in chapter 11.

However, some people will need to add a small quantity of animal protein *throughout* the two weeks of the Liver Enhancement.

A quick way to tell if you need more protein is by cravings for protein, dizziness, fatigue, lightheadedness, lethargy or feeling extra cold. If you experience any of these symptoms, even during the first two to three days, simply add 10 grams of protein (fish or eggs) per day—not per meal— and continue to add more protein until the symptoms resolve.

Digestive Bloating and Fatigue

Through surveys, we found a small percentage of the people who did this program got more bloating from adding raw vegetables. Their digestive systems had lost the ability to make the enzymes that break down these complex carbohydrates, resulting in bloating, cramps and gas. If this happens, even within the first few days, you have two choices: the first is to take a specific enzyme as a supplement;* the second is to go directly to the Adrenal/Ovary plan and consume fewer gas-producing vegetables—artichokes, asparagus, beans, broccoli, Brussels sprouts, cabbage, carrots, cauliflower, cucumbers, green beans, green peppers, lettuce, onions, radishes, sprouts and water chestnuts. This is limiting but workable. Make a log of when you eat and how you feel afterwards so you

---

* See "Enzymes to Help with Digestion" on page 314 in the resources section.

can rule out things that do not digest and avoid them for now.

Another small percentage did not have sensitivities to vegetables; they had weaknesses within their blood sugar control. Not having any animal protein made them tired and sluggish. If this occurs, start adding a little bit of protein daily (for example, an egg) and continue to add more until you feel much better. Each person's body is different and weighs more or less, so you have to determine the right amount for you.

General Overview

This short program is not so much a detoxification/cleansing process as it is a healing process to restore liver function. A healthy liver can greatly enhance weight loss.

The bulk of the foods should be raw nutrient-dense, high-fiber vegetables, minus sugars, refined foods, refined fats (trans fats), and starchy foods like potatoes.

In chapter 2, I mentioned anticancer foods would be the healthiest and would bring you to a state of health the fastest. That is why this first step includes the cruciferous family of vegetables, as they have anticancer properties (enzymes that detoxify potential carcinogens). Sprouts— especially the cruciferous type like broccoli—are one of the most nutrient-dense foods around, loaded with huge quantities of enzyme activity and anticancer factors. As a matter of fact, these sprouts have been found to contain 10–100 times the anticancer properties of mature broccoli. Omega 3 fats (flax oil, walnuts and fish oil) also have anticancer properties. Nuts and seeds are loaded with nutrition as well, but they need to be raw and germinated (soaked overnight), as you will learn in this chapter.

You can have some fruits but only an amount equal to one-third of the total vegetables you eat. You will be drinking three 8 oz cranberry drinks each day. You will also take a concentrated greens supplement to build up your potassium reserves and improve liver function. You'll be eating apples between meals and plenty of raw nuts, with some other fruits and beans. You will keep animal proteins out of the program unless your blood sugars get too low, in which case you'll need to add a small amount each day.

Food Intake

You can eat the vegetables listed below in unlimited quantities. Other vegetables not listed are also okay.

Unlimited Vegetables

- alfalfa sprouts
- artichokes
- asparagus
- avocado
- bamboo shoots
- beans
- beets
- bok choy*
- broccoli*
- Brussels sprouts*
- cabbage*
- carrots
- cauliflower*
- celery
- cilantro
- collard greens*

- corn (some)
- cucumbers
- dill
- eggplant
- escarole
- garlic
- ginger root
- kale*
- leeks
- lettuce
- mushrooms
- okra
- olives
- onions
- parsley
- peas

- peppers (all)
- pickles (w/out sugar)
- radishes*
- salsa (w/out sugar)
- sauerkraut
- seaweed
- spinach
- squash
- string beans
- sugar snap peas
- Swiss chard
- tomatoes†
- turnip greens*
- turnips*
- water chestnuts
- zucchini

○ **If you are on thyroid medication, add some foods containing iodine.** The vegetables in the above chart marked with an asterisk are cruciferous and they have a very slight effect of reducing iodine, which is used by the thyroid to make its hormones. This would probably only occur if you ate cruciferous vegetables exclusively, since raw nuts and other foods put back the iodine. But, to be conservative, if you are consuming a moderate to large quantity of cruciferous vegetables every day, add some sea kelp or

---

* Cruciferous: These are a group of vegetables belonging to the cabbage family, named for their tiny cross-shaped flowers.

† Tomatoes are really classified as fruit.

dulse to your diet—just a small sprinkle on your food or greens. Another option is alfalfa, which you can eat in food (alfalfa sprouts) or supplement form a few times a week. Alfalfa is also supplied in the Organic Cruciferous Food tablets recommended later in this chapter. So, if you choose this product for the Liver Enhancement, you will not have to worry about adding iodine when consuming cruciferous vegetables.

I recommend eating as many cruciferous vegetables as possible because of their great ability to improve the liver. The liver is the central hub for all fat-burning hormones.

○ **Kale** is a superior vegetable. This vegetable is my personal favorite, and I use raw kale as my salad greens on a daily basis. Because it is slightly bitter, I add half a raw beet, broccoli sprouts, sliced peaches and some dressing, with chopped almonds and walnuts on top.

Kale is one of the best sources of calcium, potassium, manganese and vitamins A and C. It is excellent for the liver and digestive organs. It contains cancer-fighting substances called indoles, which activate detoxifying enzymes in the liver that help neutralize potentially carcinogenic substances. Studies have shown that the plant chemicals in the kale family have a protective effect against the risk of cataracts.*

○ One ounce of **broccoli sprouts** contains the same amount of cancer-fighting properties as 1¼ pounds of cooked broccoli. In fact, Johns Hopkins University obtained the patents on one brand of broccoli sprouts after doing research on cancer.†

When a seed starts growing as a sprout, a tremendous amount of nutrition is released from that seed. If your goal is to get healthy and heal the body, sprouts are essential in your diet. Eating small quantities of sprouts is equivalent to eating large quantities of vegetables as far as nutrients are concerned. If you don't like or can't eat a lot of vegetables, then add some daily sprouts to your diet. Put them in your salad each day. You can grow them in a sprouting jar; they are also readily available in health food stores and supermarkets. Don't underestimate these tiny little greens.

○ **The vegetables may be lightly steamed.** However, it is recommended that you eat at least 50 percent of them completely raw.

---

* Source: George Mateljan Foundation, *The World's Healthiest Foods*: Kale.

† Source: Brassica Protection Products.

○ **The key is to eat as many of these vegetables as you can,** including between meals. Because they are chock-full of nutrition, it is impossible to overeat.

Dairy

Do not drink milk or consume cream cheese or sour cream. You can include a small amount (6 oz per day) of low-fat cottage cheese or plain low-fat yogurt within this plan; a little butter is okay too. Every other day you could also eat some low-fat cheese (no more than 3 oz per day), and a small quantity of feta cheese can be sprinkled on your salad as well.

An excellent breakfast could include

- ½ to 1 cup of organic low-fat cottage cheese or organic low-fat plain yogurt
- 1 teaspoon of flax oil
- ½ cup of organic fresh or frozen berries (blueberries, strawberries, etc.), or ½ cup of fresh or frozen peaches or similar fruit, or ½ teaspoon of honey (if you can't stand the taste)

If the fruit is frozen, you might want to add a bit of water before you blend the mixture. This gives you some quality protein and excellent omega 3 fats.

Don't Eat Starches

Don't eat starchy vegetables, such as French fries, baked potatoes, mashed potatoes, yams and sweet potatoes. Use corn only in very small quantities.

Don't Eat Grains

Don't consume breads, pasta, cereal, crackers, biscuits, waffles, muffins, pancakes, rice, rice cakes, donuts, etc., as they readily turn into sugar.

Allergies and Food Sensitivities

Some people are sensitive to sulfur-based vegetables like broccoli. Others are allergic to peanuts. Avoid any foods you are sensitive to. If you are experiencing bloating or gas, you need to consume only vegetables that give you no reaction. If you seem to get bloating with all vegetables, you should take an enzyme supplement or go directly to the Adrenal/Ovary plan and eat fewer gas-producing vegetables.

Salad Dressings

If you use dressing on your salad, go light on the quantity; apply it sparingly (just enough to flavor the salad) and, if at all possible, use low-sugar, natural and organic. Try to buy dressing that contains no added sugar or food colorings. Just read the labels and avoid high-fructose corn syrup, dextrose and sugar cane. Raw honey in very small amounts is an acceptable substitute. Monosodium glutamate (MSG), also known as modified food starch, must be avoided.

The health food store is your best bet. Several recommendations are Giant's Nature's Promise, Annie's Naturals, 365 Organic and Organic Ville. As a simple alternative, mix balsamic vinegar and olive oil, or even apple cider vinegar and olive oil, as a dressing.

Tip: Turmeric spice is also recommended for sprinkling on your vegetables. Studies have shown that the combination of this spice with cruciferous vegetables had significant tumor-fighting effects on certain cancers.* I sprinkle it on my salad (kale leaves), or I take cut cauliflower and either steam it or slightly cook it in coconut oil until yellow, then add turmeric on top.

Fruits

Fruits (see list on the following page) should mostly be eaten at night, with the exception of apples, which can be eaten anytime and in as much quantity as you desire. The reason for eating fruits in the later part of the day has to do with how fast they break down and turn into sugar. People who eat too many fruits for breakfast or even at lunch tend to get tired faster and don't have as much endurance. They might also crave sweets in the evenings.

---

*   Source: George Mateljan Foundation, *The World's Healthiest Foods*: Cauliflower.

Half a cup of berries or other fruit for breakfast is acceptable if eaten with low-fat cottage cheese or low-fat plain yogurt. Of all the berries, the blueberry gives you the most nutrition. Many of my clients include half a cup of organic blueberries in their diets each day. Blueberries have unique DNA protective properties, slowing the degenerative effects of aging on the brain. They also assist in preventing the binding of carcinogens to your DNA. Other recommended berries are strawberries, raspberries and elderberries.

- apples
- apricots
- berries (all)
- cherries (tart red)
- grapefruit
- grapes (red & purple)
- kiwis
- lemons/limes
- melons
- nectarines
- oranges
- peaches
- pears
- persimmons
- pineapples*
- plums
- tomatoes†

Eat only a third as many fruits, berries and melons per day as total vegetables (for example: one cup of vegetables—one-third cup of fruit).

There is a chemical in grapefruit that increases the potency of medications; so if you are taking medication, avoid grapefruits and grapefruit juice.

Even though all fruits are sweet, some have higher fiber content, which slows the absorption of sugar.

The best fruit is the **apple**.

○ High in malic acid—a good solvent for stagnant bile in the liver.
○ Pectin (gelatinous substance found in apples) helps with cardiovascular and digestive health.
○ May lower incidence of cancer.
○ In its whole form, it is high in fiber and slows insulin response.
○ High in potassium and contains no sodium.

Don't eat the following fruits, as they have extra sugar content with lower fiber: bananas, dates, figs, raisins, canned fruits, dried fruits and mangoes. And definitely avoid juices. The fiber in the whole fruit buffers the fat-making hormone insulin.

---

* Small amounts.

† Also in vegetable category.

Animal Proteins

Do not eat animal proteins (meat, chicken, etc.) or fish in the first two weeks. However, if by the second or third day you are feeling lightheaded or dizzy, or experience brain fog, fatigue and/or overall body cold due to low blood sugar, or if you notice some hair loss or have cravings for protein, add a small amount of animal protein each day.

With this program, you are consuming lots of greens, low or little fat and minimal animal protein. Since fat readily satisfies hunger and this program is low in fat, in order to avoid hunger you need to compensate by eating more food more frequently. The most important action is to eat enough food to keep your calories up, as low calories will add stress and more weight gain. That is why it's imperative that you eat between meals. In parts of this book, if you are a Liver type, I recommend only three meals per day. Nevertheless, when you are on this Liver Enhancement Plan, I want you to eat between meals as well.

If you need to eat animal proteins, as mentioned above, the following are the acceptable and preferred proteins:

Fish (wild-caught)	Grass-Fed	Eggs
Tuna, salmon,	Organic Meats	(free-range
cod, etc.—baked,	Buffalo, beef,	organic)
not deep fried;	lamb, etc.	
sashimi/sushi (without rice)		

Start with one egg per day (it could be hard-boiled) or a small piece of fish. The raw fish in sashimi and sushi is ideal.

Do not overeat animal proteins—eat just the right amount to satisfy your hunger. It's better to eat frequent small amounts, since overeating will stress the liver and convert protein to fat. Fish is the best protein on this program, and raw proteins are more easily digested, causing less liver stress.

Raw Nuts and Seeds

You'll need to eat an ample amount of raw nuts and seeds between meals to prevent hunger. Raw almonds and walnuts are best. Hummus (chickpeas) is another possibility. Some people could be allergic to nuts or will experience bloating if the nuts and seeds are not germinated (soaked overnight in water), and on the next page I will explain how to do this.

- Almonds
- Cashews*
- Hazelnuts
- Hummus
- Pecans
- Pine nuts
- Pistachios
- Pumpkin seeds
- Sesame seeds
- Sunflower seeds
- Walnuts

- Peanut butter mixed with tahini butter (raw sesame seeds)

Walnuts:
- Highest omega 3 fatty acids of any nut.
- Nutrient-dense to help satiety (feeling full).
- Decrease bad cholesterol (LDL).
- Nutritional factors in walnuts may prevent cancer cell growth.
- Can help patients with type 2 diabetes.†

Roasted nuts, like peanuts, create the biggest problem in larger quantities, and raw peanuts just don't taste good. You could have fewer peanuts and small amounts of peanut butter, providing you eat raw nuts as well and make sure the peanut butter doesn't contain added sugar or hydrogenated oils. I like dipping sliced apples in a mixture of 50 percent peanut butter and 50 percent tahini (sesame seed) butter.

Nuts and seeds grow into trees and plants. Enzymes within them activate this growth (enzymes are substances that cause and increase the speed of chemical reactions). However, inherently, nuts and seeds also have what are called *enzyme inhibitors*, which are tiny locks that prevent growth. *Inhibit* means "to hold back or keep from some action," and enzyme inhibitors keep enzyme activity from happening until the right condition exists for the nut or seed to grow into a tree or plant capable of reproduction. The main element that establishers this right condition for growth is water.

Sometimes consuming nuts and seeds in sufficient quantity can cause unpleasant heaviness in the abdomen, even bloating and gas. This is because

---

* Consume very small amounts, as many people have difficulty digesting these nuts.

† Sources: Loma Linda University 2005; Walnut Marketing Board 2005.

of the enzyme inhibitors. In other words, eating nuts and seeds without first inactivating their enzyme inhibitors forces the pancreas to work overtime, releasing lots of its *own* enzymes. A stressed pancreas will slow digestion and cause bloating. When this happens over an extended period of time, you start to lose your enzyme reserves and, without all of your enzymes, you'll have a hard time digesting foods like cruciferous vegetables. People mistake this condition for an allergy to the cruciferous vegetables. Studies performed on animals that were fed nuts with enzyme inhibitors in tact showed a doubling in size of the animals' pancreases, stunted growth, impaired health and decreased enzyme reserves.

So, how do we handle this problem?

Squirrels bury their nuts in the ground to activate the enzymes and deactivate the enzyme inhibitors. (That's one thing you could do, but first let me get my camera!) You could also cook the nuts and seeds, although the heat would destroy the nutritional value, since enzymes are very sensitive to any heat. This is why you should consume raw nuts rather than roasted nuts. The best thing to do is activate the enzymes in the nuts and seeds to start the process of germination (*germinate* means "to cause to sprout or grow"). Here is the way you do this:

1. Soak your seeds and nuts in filtered or spring water overnight—12 hours is ideal—in a covered glass or metal container. Cheesecloth makes a good cover.

2. In the morning, rinse the seeds and nuts several times to drain off the fluid containing the enzyme inhibitors.

3. Let them dry on some surface like a wire strainer that will let air permeate. You might find that they stay moist, which is fine as long as you keep them in the refrigerator until you eat them. It is best to soak only the quantity of seeds and nuts you will eat within 4 to 5 days, because soaking makes them more "alive" and more susceptible to spoiling. If you can't eat them within that time, you could use a dehydrator to remove all the water; set it at 105 degrees F (not more because, remember, the good enzymes are sensitive to too much heat) for 18–24 hours.

4. Start eating. You are now consuming live superfood. This process of germination will not only take stress off your digestive system, it will

also increase the availability of additional active enzymes, vitamins, and minerals such as calcium, magnesium, iron, copper and zinc.

5. Store what you don't eat in a glass container in your refrigerator to increase shelf life and freshness, as germinated seeds and nuts do not keep as long.

Beans/Lentils

You could add beans/lentils to this program as well. Refried beans and baked beans are not recommended. Before you cook beans, you'll need to soak them in water overnight, just as you should do with nuts and seeds. This allows them to release their enzyme inhibitors so that they will digest better and contain maximum nutrition. A great way to get more nutrients from beans and lentils is to sprout them. However, never sprout kidney beans, as these must be fully cooked, otherwise they can cause digestive upset.

Many Indian dishes include heavily cooked lentils and beans. The more overcooked something is, the less nutrition it has and the more stress there is on the liver. The more stress on the liver, the less weight you will lose.

Supplement Intake

There is one type of supplement recommended. It is a special greens product. This nutrient will supply the raw material for the liver to rejuvenate as well as build up your cells' potassium reserves.

It is difficult to find quality greens products, let alone one containing cruciferous greens, so I personally created a high-quality organic cruciferous food concentrate with several additional vegetables for other health benefits. It's called **Organic Cruciferous Food**. It contains organic asparagus, alfalfa grass juice, beets, broccoli, Brussels sprouts, cabbage, cauliflower, celery, collard greens, kale, parsley, radish and spinach.

Many of my patients take this product to supplement their diets, as they don't always include in their meals the cruciferous family of vegetables. There are some big advantages to using cruciferous vegetables over just greens, a principal one being they are very beneficial for the liver. A lot of people don't eat or don't like eating these vegetables, but the ironic thing is if they did eat them, they wouldn't be reading this book.

There is another high-quality acceptable supplement that you may choose to take in place of the Organic Cruciferous Food. The Standard Process purification and weight management programs utilize several greens products, which are recommended by many healthcare practitioners to their patients. Standard Process has been my main source of whole-food supplements for years, and these two programs include a cruciferous greens product along with several others that benefit the body. If you decide to use these supplements, you'll need to find a practitioner in your area who carries Standard Process products.*

Recommended Supplement

Organic Cruciferous Food — 15 per day. The dosage can be split up into three times per day or smaller amounts more frequently throughout the day.

Don't be shocked at this dosage, as you are only eating concentrated food. The purpose of these specific foods is to, as quickly as possible, balance the fluids in your body and improve liver function. Cruciferous vegetables are extremely high in potassium and low in sodium, so they help to balance the fluids and slow the insulin fat-making response. The other advantage of this supplement is that it contains alfalfa grass juice, which has iodine.

After the Liver Enhancement phase, which could last two weeks or significantly longer, a good maintenance product called **Organic Cruciferous Sprouts Food** is recommended, especially if you do not consume sprouts in your diet. This is a blend of seven organic cruciferous freeze-dried sprouts, with no binders of any kind. (For more information, see Organic Cruciferous Food on page 333.)†

---

* See the entry for Standard Process Inc. on page 315 in the resources section.

† To order Organic Cruciferous Food and Organic Cruciferous Sprouts Food, see page 314 in the resources section.

Cranberry Drink

You will be drinking a mixture containing unsweetened cranberry juice, lemon and apple cider vinegar.

This mixture should be taken three times per day (three 8 oz glasses):
1. first thing in the morning upon rising
2. before lunch
3. before dinner

Ingredients

- Spring water (6 oz).
- Unsweetened cranberry juice (2 oz or ¼ of a glass); make sure you read the label, as many people purchase the sweetened cranberry juice by mistake. Even though pure cranberry juice is very bitter, it does contain around 8 grams of sugar per 6 ounces. This is usually okay. The type of cranberry juice you do not want to use is the cranberry mixed with apple juice and other juices, bringing the sugar levels up to 28 grams per 6 ounces. Do not be concerned if your cranberry juice is not organic, as it is very difficult to find organic cranberry juice. For those people who have major struggles with losing even a little weight, I recommend omitting cranberry juice from this mixture, since just a minute amount of sugar can potentially block fat burning.
- Lemon juice—⅓ of a fresh lemon or 1 tsp of lemon powder. If you have a history of kidney stones, use a whole lemon or 3 tsp of lemon powder. Both the cranberry juice and eating a grapefruit each day will also help prevent kidney stones.
- Apple cider vinegar (½ to 1 tsp); adjust amount to your taste, as this might be too strong for some people.
- Apple juice—only use if the drink is unpalatable (maximum amount is ¼ cup). But, if possible, omit apple juice, as it is concentrated sugar.
- OPTION: A certain percentage of my patients like to add some fiber to this drink. I have observed that people are less hungry when they add fiber. This could be any type of psyllium seed or husk or other powdered fiber. Two tablespoons would be enough.

It is recommended that you mix the entire combination together in a container the night before and place it in the refrigerator or a cooler. If you absolutely cannot stand this drink mixture, don't force yourself to drink it. I have found most people love it and a few hate it. Some bodies just can't tolerate the vinegar; so, there is some flexibility in drinking the mixture without the vinegar.

Purpose of Ingredients

Unsweetened Cranberry Juice

This juice helps support normal kidney, bladder and urinary tract functions—the body's filtration system. It is very high in potassium and low in sodium. Since the liver and kidneys work together, they both need to be supported. This juice can be found at any health food store. You can use powdered cranberry as well—go to http://www.usjuice.com/ and click on "Unsweetened Cranberry Powder."

Lemon Juice

Lemons support normal immune function. Lemon juice also helps contract the liver (astringent). You can use one-third of a real lemon or one teaspoon of lemon powder.

Apple Cider Vinegar

I would recommend Bragg apple cider vinegar; however, any brand will work. There are many benefits, including balancing the pH of the body, eliminating waste acids and providing potassium, as well as fortifying the friendly bacteria in your intestines. It helps reduce water retention through the normalization of acid and alkaline levels.

A Few Guidelines

1. Refrain from eating anything that is not on the lists given in this Liver Enhancement Plan. This especially includes sugar and hidden sugars — juice, sports drinks, protein bars, vanilla yogurt, etc. Consume walnuts, as they are a superior nut.

2. You can drink as much water and herbal tea as you desire, but only drink the amount of water you are thirsty for. Don't ever force yourself to drink too much water. Green tea (naturally decaffeinated) is another option.

3. Avoid drinking tap water. Spring water is best. Filtered water is okay.

4. Avoid coffee during this phase. If you find this is impossible, gradually cut down and mix decaffeinated coffee for one to two weeks until you are weaned off. Coming off coffee cold turkey will create lethargy for about one to two days. If possible, use organic coffee.

5. This Liver Enhancement Plan can be done every other month to keep the liver in top shape. Some people continue the Liver Enhancement for months until they start craving protein, at which point they introduce an adequate amount to turn off the craving.

6. The exercise program can be combined when doing this Liver Enhancement Plan, but only if your energy is high; and make sure you keep your pulse rate low, below 130.

7. Avoid dairy. A small amount of low-fat cottage cheese or plain low-fat yogurt is acceptable, also a little butter and low-fat cheese.

8. Avoid anything with MSG (monosodium glutamate). MSG is a flavor enhancer, which not only makes the food taste better than it is but makes you hungrier. This is why you can't stop eating just one potato chip, and this is also why you get hungry one hour after consuming Chinese food. Many restaurant foods, especially Chinese, contain this chemical. It is a big fluid retainer.

Three-Day Sample of 14-Day Enhancement Plan

Monday

Breakfast
Cranberry Drink + Greens Product
- Cut vegetables with raw nuts
- Apple dipped in peanut butter

Midmorning Snack
- Raw nuts/seeds

Lunch
Cranberry Drink + Greens Product
- Salad with almonds, kale, red cabbage and black olives
- 1 apple

Afternoon Snack
- 1 apple

Dinner
Cranberry Drink + Greens Product
- Kidney beans
- Hummus
- Avocado

Evening Snack
- Black olives and pickles

Tuesday

Breakfast
Cranberry Drink + Greens Product
- ½ cup low-fat cottage cheese or plain low-fat yogurt
- 1 teaspoon of flax oil
- ½ cup of berries or other fruit

Midmorning Snack
- 1 apple

Lunch
Cranberry Drink + Greens Product
- Asparagus + butter
- Sliced cucumbers
- 1 apple + raw nuts

Afternoon Snack
- Grapefruit

Dinner
Cranberry Drink + Greens Product
- Fruit salad + raw nuts
- Coleslaw

Evening Snack
- Bowl of berries

Three-Day Sample of 14-Day Enhancement Plan

Wednesday

Breakfast

Cranberry Drink + Greens Product
- Sautéed mushrooms
  with onions
- Raw pecans

Midmorning Snack

- Peanut butter with celery

Lunch

Cranberry Drink + Greens Product
- Green pepper, steamed broccoli
  with butter
- 1 apple + raw almonds

Afternoon Snack

- Celery and carrot sticks with nuts

Dinner

Cranberry Drink + Greens Product
- Cauliflower sautéed in butter or
  coconut oil until slightly brown +
  mixed green salad

Evening Snack

- Raw nuts

Quick Healthy Small Meals & Snacks

- Button mushrooms sautéed in butter
- Apple slices dipped in peanut butter
- Plain low-fat yogurt with added pecans
- Bran Crispbread* with peanut butter
- Cut vegetables dipped in guacamole (avocado, onion, tomato, cumin, mayonnaise, lemon juice and garlic)
- Pickles and olives (for people who crave salt)
- Cooked cabbage with garlic and onion
- Bran Crispbread with low-fat cheese (3 oz)
- Cut apple in hummus (chickpeas, garlic, lemon juice and tahini butter)
- Cucumber slices in dill dip
- Plain low-fat yogurt (6 oz) with apple sauce
- Bran Crispbread with hummus
- Celery dipped in a mixture of peanut butter and tahini butter (sesame seeds)
- Spaghetti squash with tomato sauce (low sugar)
- Plain low-fat yogurt (6 oz) with cut pineapple
- Plain low-fat yogurt (6 oz) with berries
- Low-fat cheese melted over broccoli
- Fried eggplant (in olive oil)
- Slightly cooked cauliflower with turmeric spice
- Tomato and basil leaf with low-fat cheese (3 oz)

---

* For more information, see page 314 in the resources section.

Salad Ideas

- Tomato, avocado, black pepper, basil leaves, sprouts
- Cabbage (shredded), pineapple chunks, almonds, kale
- Steamed or pickled beets, cucumbers, onion (sautéed)
- Lettuce, apple, lemon juice, kidney beans, sprouts
- Chickpeas, romaine lettuce, black olives
- Bok choy, asparagus, sugar snap peas, carrots, sunflower seeds
- Cabbage, celery, parsley, cashews, sprouts
- Steamed spinach, peas, ginger root, lentils, lime juice
- Pinto beans, tomatoes, avocado, olives, red cabbage
- Cabbage, sautéed mushrooms, cauliflower sautéed in butter or coconut oil until slightly brown
- Cauliflower sautéed in butter or coconut oil until slightly brown, spinach, carrots, broccoli
- Cauliflower sautéed in butter or coconut oil until slightly brown, hummus
- Black-eyed peas, kidney beans, bell pepper, onion, parsley
- Red cabbage, cut pears, shredded carrots, cut apple
- Green pepper, cucumbers, carrots, kale, sprouts
- Broccoli with ranch dip, artichoke hearts
- Cut apple, black olives, celery, lemon juice, mayonnaise
- Lettuce, honeydew melon, strawberries, mint leaf
- Baby spinach, sprouts, celery, beets (raw, not canned)
- Kale, papaya, avocado, apple, black olives

Concentrated Nutrition

There are receptors in your digestive system that signal the brain and tell it when to feel hungry and when to be satisfied. When you consume highly concentrated nutrients, the body's hunger centers are easily satisfied, resulting in fewer cravings and less hunger. This is why you can eat a lot of refined "empty nutrition" bread or other carbohydrate, since carbohydrates do not trigger the brain hunger centers as readily. The reason your cravings will go away on this program is because the body is getting all the nutrition it needs. Cravings only occur when you are missing some nutrients.

What to Expect

At the end of the two-week program, you should notice that your cravings are gone, your bowel movements should be improved, your energy should be up, and you should be losing weight and/or inches. About 20 percent of my patients didn't lose much weight during this initial cleanse (only five pounds) for two reasons: (1) their body was healing and needed more time to regenerate muscle protein, or (2) they were an Adrenal or Ovary body type and required more protein. However, just about everyone will experience improved energy, better sleep, fewer cravings, and improvements in hair, nails, skin and sex drive because of the liver's enhanced ability to utilize hormones. People who have fluid weight can lose pounds faster than those with actual fat as weight. Normalization of blood pressure and cholesterol can also be noticed. This is due to the improved liver function. If you are taking medication and these changes occur, get with your doctor so that he or she can adjust the dosage.

It's important to know that water weight comes off before fat weight. This means you might initially lose lots of weight and then it will slow down when you get into fat burning. Many people get discouraged by this and think the program is not working. It is working. You just have to know that two pounds of fat loss is the maximum possible per week. The determining factor in exactly how much fat is lost will be the level of health of your glands. The worse off the metabolism, the more closely you need to follow the diet.

What Will You Do after the Two Weeks?

At the end of 14 days, you have to make a decision whether to stay on this program longer or start adding some protein. If the liver has been in bad shape, it will take some time to bring it back. Don't expect the liver to regenerate in two weeks; this is just the beginning. Some of my patients do the Liver Enhancement every two months.

If you experienced excellent results during the two weeks and feel like you could go longer, I would recommend continuing as long as you can. Why change a successful action? Some people stay on it an additional one to three weeks and others continue for several months, while some are ready to come off it after 14 days, as they are craving a steak. Your body will let you know when it needs more protein.

For example, a patient came in with a huge abdomen and did the 14-day Liver Enhancement, lost 15 pounds and decreased cholesterol and blood pressure. His energy and sleep were great, not to mention improved bowel function. He then stopped the Liver Enhancement and started with more protein. His results worsened. I told him to go back on the Liver Enhancement and ride the wave as long as he could. He did and continued it for another two months, losing his excess stomach. He then added a small amount of protein and continued to lose weight.

What's Next?

Now that you have completed the Liver Enhancement, you are ready for step two. So, turn to the next chapter.

11

Step TWO:
What to Eat Next

You should have now completed the Liver Enhancement Plan and be ready for step two—the Maintenance Plan.

One of the challenges is finding out what body type you have. It's not always black and white. It might be mixed. You might have a little bit of this and a little bit of that. So, rather than lock you into ONE body type and ONE diet, we will find out what body type you have, based on how your body responds to food. Once you discover what works best for you, you'll want to maintain those foods.

All four body types need the same key basic healing foods. However, the amount of protein and fat will vary. Because different body types (Adrenal, Ovary, Thyroid and Liver) need different amounts of protein, you will add more protein based on how your body responds to the initial phase. This change (additional protein) will be done gradually until you find the right amount. If your body responds better to high-vegetable, low-protein foods (Liver Enhancement or Liver & Thyroid types), don't change anything. If your weakness is within the adrenals or ovaries, you will need more protein in the diet. And with protein comes more fat, since they are usually together as foods.

The strategy is to find out what gives you the best overall improvement. However, since weight loss is just *one* indicator of improvement, we will look at all six additional factors.

The way you will judge or know when to start adding more protein will be by feedback from ALL seven of these body changes:

1. Energy level
2. Sleep quality
3. Amount of sleep
4. Cravings
5. Overall digestion
6. Inches lost
7. Weight lost

To find the correct amount of protein you need, you will start at the left on the chart below and move to the right. In other words, you will be adjusting your eating to find out what diet will give you the maximum energy, best quality sleep, the least cravings, and the best overall digestion. These things tell you if the program is working. If these factors are high, the weight comes off as a result.

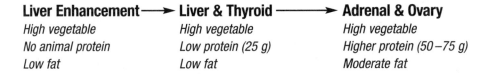

Liver Enhancement———▶ **Liver & Thyroid** ————————▶ **Adrenal & Ovary**
High vegetable   *High vegetable*   *High vegetable*
No animal protein   *Low protein (25 g)*   *Higher protein (50 – 75 g)*
Low fat   *Low fat*   *Moderate fat*

You will only move to the right and add more protein if you have low energy, poor sleep, cravings, poor digestion and no inch or weight loss. Low energy includes moodiness, irritability, lethargy or depression. However, if you are having positive changes with the Liver Enhancement Plan (high vegetable, no animal protein and low fat), you will continue what worked. I have found the majority of people get the best results with very little protein. A smaller percentage will lose more weight on higher amounts of protein and fat, or somewhere in between.

Remember your goal is to GET HEALTHY so that your body can burn fat. Getting healthy requires an initial healing phase, which might not show up at first in weight loss, but will show up as improvement in these other factors—energy, sleep, cravings, digestion, and inches lost. Depending on what's happening with your body, you may need more or less protein for this phase.

Basic Rules of Eating for Hormone Health

Essential Rules and Examples

Avoid sugar, sweet fruits, grains and starches

Avoid sweeteners, candy, juice, and sugar in yogurt (vanilla too). The only acceptable sweeteners in very small amounts are stevia, raw honey, Tupelo honey or agave nectar—but it's recommended to avoid these until you achieve significant weight loss.

Avoid sweet fruits—bananas, dates, figs, raisins, mangoes, canned fruits and dried fruits. You can have higher fiber fruits and berries but only one-third of the amount of vegetables you eat.

Avoid grains—breads, pasta, crackers, cereal and others. Oatmeal and brown rice are less damaging but should be consumed only once per week.

Avoid starches—potatoes, yams and corn. Red potatoes are the least damaging but should be eaten only once per week (small amount), if at all.

Consume lots of raw, whole, nutrient-dense, high-fiber vegetables

This includes all the nonstarchy vegetables, salads, leafy greens, cruciferous, etc. Eat them in their whole form and preferably raw (at least 50 percent). If you are a true Thyroid type, add sea kelp, dulse or alfalfa for extra iodine. You can consume beans/lentils, but avoid refried or baked beans. Eating vegetables with each meal is recommended. You can use salad dressings and dips without MSG and without excessive sugar.

Don't allow yourself to get hungry

Because you are eating lots of vegetables that are low in fat, you might feel hungrier. This means you need to **eat more and between meals**. However, if you are mainly a Liver type, it is recommended that you eat only three meals per day with no snacking in between. Do not skip a meal or let yourself get hungry. Compensate by eating more green vegetables.

Consume the right amount of protein for your body type

Start out with small quantities of protein per day. Depending on the seven indicators, you will slowly add more protein until you achieve your optimum amount. Eat grass-fed animal products and wild-caught fish. Avoid protein powders, protein bars, pasteurized milk and too much cooked protein, especially overly cooked protein.

Consume the right balance and amount of fat for your body type

Start out with low fats — low-fat cottage cheese, low-fat cheese, low-fat yogurt. Avoid hydrogenated and partially hydrogenated fats (trans fats). Avocados, olives and raw nuts are okay. As you progress, you will add more fats (butter, sour cream, cream cheese, whole-milk yogurt, etc.); but if you start getting bloated (digestive), fatigued, experience sleeplessness and have right shoulder pain, cut them back, as some people with poor livers cannot digest/tolerate fats and oils. The right amounts include a 1:1:1 ratio of saturated fats to unsaturated omega 3 (fish/flax oil) and omega 6 (vegetables, raw nuts, seeds, olives or olive oil) essential fats.

Avoid gland blockers

Avoid caffeinated beverages and foods (coffee, soda, sports drinks, diet pills, energy drinks and chocolate).

Eat at least 50 percent organic and hormone-free foods. Avoid packaged or boxed foods with lots of chemicals. Avoid soy products, which are usually genetically modified.

If you are on medications, you need to compensate and eat even more raw vegetables (cruciferous and beets are best).

Avoid water retainers

Avoid anything with MSG, including hidden sources under other names. Monosodium glutamate is abundant in many restaurant foods, taco mixes, sauces, gravies, boxed foods, soups and dressings. Read the labels.

Avoid artificial sweeteners, such as high-fructose corn syrup, dextrose, glucose and sugar alcohols (including Splenda).

Refined carbohydrates/sugar can deplete your body of potassium and retain sodium — avoid them.

Exercise for your body type

We will discuss this in the chapter on exercise, as it's best to do the eating plan first so that you have more energy to exercise. I don't recommend exercising if you are tired — this is especially true for the Adrenal type. In fact, many people who have adrenal weakness gain weight with exercise.

Reduce stress

Do your best to reduce stress; you will be amazed how better eating will drop your stress level. One counter to stress is exercise — especially low-pulse-rate walking. Pain and inflammation in the body can keep you out of fat burning because of high levels of cortisol. Seek help for pain. Of course, I'm a little biased and recommend my acupressure technique for this.*

Get an adequate amount of sleep

As you clean up your diet and follow this program to find the foods you respond to best, sleep should improve greatly. Get to bed before 11:00 p.m. Many people who eat poorly (especially sweets) will have digestive bloating, which will keep them from sleeping. A sick body can't get deep quality sleep. Try to get at least **seven hours per night**.

---

* For more information, see the glossary, page 283, and the resources section, page 313.

Other Tips on Eating for Hormone Health

1. As you increase protein, *space out proteins evenly throughout the day*, eating smaller amounts with each meal rather than a large amount all at one time. You need to eat whole protein, not processed protein (powders and bars). Your body can only digest a certain amount of protein per meal and anything over that adds more stress — you should never feel bloated after a meal. Overeating protein can turn it to fat. The chart on the next page shows the amount of protein you need.

2. *Do not skip meals.* Snack on nuts, seeds and apples through the day. Because fats are low, you might experience more hunger. This is why you need to eat between meals to prevent hunger. Night snacking should be fewer nuts/seeds and more either vegetables or fruits — celery, carrots, grapefruit or apple. If you find out you are more of a Liver type, you will eat only three meals per day and not snack between meals.

3. If you are going to consume berries or fruit, *eat the majority in the evening* (after 5:00 p.m.), not for breakfast. This will keep the fuel in your body burning more evenly. If you eat only fruits and berries for breakfast, you could end up craving sweets later in the day or at night because of lower blood sugar.

The results of the initial program will give valuable feedback as to what eating plan you should continue. The great majority of people (60 percent) will get the most success (weight loss, increased energy, etc.) with the Liver Enhancement. Around 30 percent will do best on the Adrenal & Ovary eating plan. The rest will fit somewhere in between. Once you find your program, stick with it until you achieve your weight and health goals. At that point your body will adapt to this lifestyle and you will want to continue it, and your metabolism will have stabilized.

In the next section, I've given you another way of looking at these overall eating plans. My intention is to make this as simple as possible.

Overview of the Different Eating Plans

Listed below are the general guidelines for Liver Enhancement and the four body types, categorized by food groups.

Proteins (animal, fish, dairy)

Liver Enhancement *(per day)*
Zero animal/fish
Avoid dairy: 6 oz of low-fat cottage cheese or plain low-fat yogurt is acceptable, as well as a little butter and some low-fat cheese (no more than 3 oz every other day); a small quantity of feta cheese can also be sprinkled over salad

Liver & Thyroid *(per day)*
~25 grams

Adrenal & Ovary *(per day)*
~50–75 grams

Nonanimal Proteins (nuts/seeds)

For Liver Enhancement as well as all four body types, eat an ample amount of nuts and seeds. If these are germinated (soaked in water overnight) they will be easier to digest. The quantity will vary from individual to individual; some will be able to eat more than others. However, if you find that nuts and seeds cause bloating, eat smaller amounts.

Vegetables .

Liver Enhancement *(per day)*
Large amount

Liver & Thyroid *(per day)*
Large amount—if a Liver type, consume lots of cruciferous vegetables; if a true Thyroid type, eat lots of noncruciferous vegetables or, if you eat cruciferous, add some sea kelp, dulse or alfalfa

Adrenal & Ovary *(per day)*
Large amount

Fats

Liver Enhancement *(per day)*
Zero to small—flax oil is okay

Liver & Thyroid *(per day)*
Small (no or low fats)—flax oil is okay

Adrenal & Ovary *(per day)*
Moderate (whole fats, not reduced); flax oil is okay

Beans/Lentils

Liver Enhancement *(per day)*
Small—less than 3 oz

Liver & Thyroid *(per day)*
Small—less than 3 oz

Adrenal & Ovary *(per day)*
Small—less than 3 oz

Fruit

Liver Enhancement *(per day)*
Small amount, equal to one-third of total vegetables, with the exception of apples, which can be consumed in unlimited quantity

Liver & Thyroid *(per day)*
Small amount, with the exception of apples, which can be consumed in unlimited quantity

Adrenal & Ovary *(per day)*
Small amount, with the exception of apples, which can be consumed in unlimited quantity

There is a chemical in grapefruit that increases the potency of medications; so if you are taking medication, avoid grapefruits and grapefruit juice. This applies to all of the eating plans.

Frequency of Eating

Liver Enhancement *(per day)*
Frequent meals with snacks

Liver & Thyroid *(per day)*
Liver: 3 meals (no snacks)
Thyroid: 3 meals with snacks

Adrenal & Ovary *(per day)*
Frequent meals with snacks

So-Called "Natural" Foods

Simply because a food product says "natural" on the label, this does not always mean what is implied. There are five things in foods that you should be aware of:

1. *Pesticides, insecticides and other chemical sprays:* Back in the 1930s we started using chemicals to decrease a 20 percent loss of crops. Presently, with the addition of thousands of new chemicals, we still have a 20 percent loss of crops.

2. *Growth hormones:* Farmers use growth hormones for one thing—to make animals grow faster and bigger.

3. *Antibiotics:* Farmers also use antibiotics to make their animals grow larger, but they are used as well to prevent infection and disease. I believe this is the reason for new strains of nearly impossible to kill microbes.

4. *Animal feed containing restaurant grease and animal waste:* Animal waste is recycled into animal feeds and hidden as "protein isolates." The FDA allows each state to regulate how animal waste is processed

and recycled back into animal feeds. It is apparently too expensive and toxic for landfills. Restaurant grease is also recycled into animal feeds. Because the waste grease from fast-food restaurants is a health hazard, these establishments are not allowed to drain their used oils and grease through the sewage system. Their cost-effective "solution" has been to recycle these oils (including harmful hydrogenated oil) and place them back into animal feeds. Animal offal (meaning waste parts from a butchered animal, garbage or rubbish) is also recycled into feeds, which includes blood, guts and feathers.*

5. *Addictive chemicals added to foods:* Many food producers put addictive chemicals in their products as a means of controlling the consumer into continuing to buy and eat their foods. Monosodium glutamate (flavor enhancer) is one of them. MSG doesn't alter the way food tastes; it increases and enhances the sensitivity of taste buds, acting like a drug to excite them. MSG tricks your brain into thinking the food tastes good. It also inhibits the sensation of being satisfied, so you continue to eat. Because of the sodium in monoSODIUM glutamate, water is retained.

Cutting out foods contaminated with antibiotics, pesticides, growth hormones and other chemicals introduced into our mainstream food supply is essential to your weight loss success as well as to your health. Therefore it is imperative to consume a good portion of organically grown foods. Organic foods are fertilized and grown without the use of toxic chemicals of any kind. It is not always practical to consume 100 percent organic all the time, but if you can eat 50 percent organic, you'll be doing well.

Sugar and Hidden Sugars

Sugar and hidden sugars are at the top of the fat-making-hormone triggers. Very small amounts of these foods will keep you fully out of fat-burning for long periods of time. In fact, the fat on your body comes from the hidden sugars, not from the fat you've been eating. Use the substitution chart on the next page to counter these temptations.

---

* Sources: Crickenberger and Carawan 1996; Kirby 1999; Research Consortium Sustainable Animal Production 2000.

Sugar, Hidden Sugars, Grains & Starches

Snacks and Desserts	Substitute
Chocolate	This could be a serotonin deficiency. Eat a small red potato with butter (sparingly, once per week) to help bring your serotonin levels up.
Candies	Low-carb candy sweetened with stevia, if any at all.
Crackers	GG Bran Crispbread (50 percent fiber, zero net carb); could be eaten anytime, since it's mostly bran (outer shell of grain): http://www.brancrispbread.com/. Crispbread (low-sugar, high-fiber rye cracker), any of the following brands: Kavli, Finn Crisp or Ryvita. These can be eaten occasionally. Go to your local health food store (e.g., Whole Foods Market).
Flour products (breads, pasta, cereal, cakes, waffles, pancakes, donuts, cookies, etc.)	Ezekiel flourless sprouted bread, pastas, cereal, tortillas, muffins, buns — use sparingly: http://www.foodforlife.com/.
Commercial white and whole-wheat breads	Spelt bread — use sparingly.
Ice cream	Homemade whipped cream (no sugar) with strawberries, berries or pineapple.
Canned fruit with syrup	Fresh pineapple. Canned pineapple is pasteurized, so enzymes are reduced.
Flavored yogurt	Plain, unsweetened yogurt mixed with applesauce or berries.
White sugar	Raw honey in small amounts. Tupelo honey or agave nectar is also fine, but it's best to avoid it altogether.
White rice	Steamed brown rice or Mochi (brown rice squares) by Grainaissance — use sparingly: http://www.grainaissance.com/.
Oatmeal (prepackaged)	Steel-cut oatmeal — use sparingly.
Sweet fruits (bananas, dates, figs, mangoes, raisins and dried fruit)	Less sweet fruits — apples, melons, pears, berries, oranges, grapefruits, etc.

Gland Blockers

The next chart will give you some substitutes for major gland blockers. Without removing the things that are destroying your endocrine system, it cannot heal.

Gland Blockers

Avoid	Substitute
Alcohol	Nonalcoholic beverages; low-carb light beer is the least damaging — use sparingly
Coffee	Water-processed organic decaffeinated coffee; another option is Teeccino, an herbal coffee, obtainable from health food stores or online at http://www.teeccino.com/
Black tea (caffeinated)	Herb tea or green tea (naturally decaffeinated)
Artificial fats	Real butter, coconut butter (small amounts)
Hydrogenated fats, margarine, Crisco and partially hydrogenated oils	Expeller-pressed oils (small amounts) — coconut, safflower, olive and peanut oils are best to cook with; on salads use flax, olive, sesame seed, sunflower and walnut oils
Deep-fried fats	Deep-fried peanut oil (sparingly)
Sharp cheese	Mild cheeses
Commercial eggs (hormone-fed chickens)	Organic eggs (hormone free, free range)
Commercial hamburger, deli meats, pork and chicken	Free-range animal meats, grass-fed or fed on pesticide-free grains and not given antibiotics or growth hormones
Meats with nitrates	Meats without nitrates
Farm-raised fish	Fresh-water or wild-caught fish (hormone free)
Overcooked beef or steak	Rare or medium-rare steak — fish is an easier-to-digest protein; Liver types do better on less red meat meals (1 to 2 times per week)
Pasteurized milk	Spring water or herb tea
Chips with partially hydrogenated oil (trans fats)	Chips from just corn or potato with peanut oil or safflower oil and preferably sea salt — use sparingly because these are starches

- "Use sparingly" means out of all the foods in this category you could have just one per week; however, it is recommended that you eliminate them altogether. The worse off your metabolism, the less you can get away with the "use sparingly" group.
- Many people think because bread is whole wheat, it is healthier and less fattening. There's not much difference in the speed at which these flour products turn into sugar and then fat. Often commercial whole-wheat bread is exposed to more chemical sprays than white bread because it has more nutrition and so attracts more pests.

Water Retainers

Avoiding water retainers is equally as important as avoiding things that destroy your hormones. You might find it challenging to avoid these high-sodium items, especially when eating out. I've included a helpful chart on the next page.

Beverages

Juices, sodas and soft drinks have high sugar content, and diet sodas and other drinks contain undesirable artificial sweeteners and/or artificial colors. In many areas, tap water isn't the best thing to drink due to the chemicals used to purify the water. Substitute these drinks with those in the right column of the Beverage Substitution Chart below.

Beverage Substitution Chart

Beverages	Substitute
Juices	Unsweetened naturally decaffeinated herb tea, spring water, and water with ½ a squeezed lemon
Gatorade	Spring water with squeezed lemon and unsweetened cranberry juice; you could also add a hint (1 tsp) of apple cider vinegar to give extra electrolytes
Tap water with high levels of chlorine	Spring water, filtered water or carbonated spring water

Water Retainers

Processed Foods	Substitute
Salad dressings with monosodium glutamate (MSG)	Salad dressings without MSG—get the ones with the least chemicals and ingredients Use olive oil and Bragg Liquid Aminos (tastes like soy sauce)
Taco seasoning, repackaged (with autolyzed yeast extract—MSG)	Homemade taco seasoning with onion, sea salt, garlic, chili peppers and paprika
Onion dips, vegetable dips, herb dips and guacamole dips with yeast extract (MSG)	Dips without MSG (go to the local health food store)
Ketchup (commercial)	Ketchup with fructose or nonsugar sweetener
Mayonnaise (commercial)	Mayonnaise from a health food store (365 is a good brand)
Chinese restaurant foods	Homemade Chinese foods with Bragg Liquid Aminos
Rich sauces like gravies	Sour cream (low fat)
Spaghetti sauce with sugar/MSG added (especially high-fructose corn syrup)	Spaghetti sauce with minimal sugar added (Muir Glen and Walnut Acres are good brands)
Dried fruits sprayed with sulfur	Whole fresh fruits
Meats with dextrose sugar or high-fructose corn syrup	Meats containing no sugars (read labels)
Soups with MSG (mostly as autolyzed yeast extract or modified food starch)	Organic soups without MSG
Artificial sweeteners (aspartame and Sweet'N Low)	Stevia, raw honey or agave nectar (small quantities)
Sugar alcohols (xylitol, mannitol, Splenda)	Stevia, raw honey or agave nectar (small quantities)

Recommended Liquids Chart

Use Most Often

Herbal tea	Filtered water
Spring water	Well water
Lemon water	Carbonated water
Green tea	Cranberry juice (unsweetened, 2 oz) mixed with glass of water

Use Sparingly

Rice milk	Organic coffee (one small cup, in the morning)
Almond milk	Milk (if you do, always use organic)

Mercury in Fish

Do not eat shark, swordfish, king mackerel or tilefish, because they contain high levels of mercury. Five of the most commonly eaten fish that are low in mercury are **shrimp, canned light tuna, salmon, pollock and catfish.** Another commonly eaten fish, albacore ("white") tuna, has more mercury than canned light tuna. So, when choosing tuna, purchase the **canned light tuna.**[*]

Eating at Social Events, Parties and Restaurants

Social events are unavoidable and you will be in situations that make it difficult to find something to eat. But here are a few tips:

✓ Eat an apple before you go.

✓ Snack on as many nuts as you can at the event.

✓ Eat something healthy (vegetables) before and after the chocolate or cake. If you consume refined sugars and carbs, potassium is

---

[*] Sources: U.S. Dept. of Health and Human Services and U.S. Environmental Protection Agency 2004.

lost, raising sodium. Wherever sodium goes, water goes. To counter the loss of potassium, you could consume high-potassium foods — leafy greens.

✓ When you eat the junk food, just don't stuff yourself, as overeating refined carbs severely increases insulin. Choose a small piece and fill up on healthier foods.

The worst restaurants to go to on this program are Chinese restaurants because most have hidden sources of monosodium glutamate (MSG). This is a huge water retainer because of massive amounts of sodium. Even if they tell you they use no extra MSG, it's in the pre-made sauces.

Italian restaurants have lots of pasta and breaded foods. Skip the bread on the table and order some fish or steak and salad. Often the steaks come in 12 and 16 ounces, which is too much to digest comfortably. Eat only 5 to 6 ounces and take the rest home.

At Mexican restaurants, order a burrito bowl (which is chicken, salsa, lettuce, cheese and sour cream) without the tortilla, refried beans or taco shell.

If you consume a potato, add more butter or sour cream to buffer the insulin response. If you eat some popcorn, add more butter to slow the insulin response. Adding fat helps slow this process.

Tell the server to bring you a burger without the bun or French fries. Add a salad instead, and in place of ketchup use mayonnaise and mustard, as ketchup contains high-fructose corn syrup.

Realize when you eat out you are consuming many different chemicals in the sauces, breading, gravy, dips, etc. Try to eat whole foods, such as fish and vegetables, meat and salad. Skip the dessert, especially if you are eating meat, as together they affect hormones negatively.

Adding a sugary dessert or alcohol to the meal puts a strain on digestion, which severely affects insulin. Even though you might be a social outcast if you avoid these, you'll feel better several hours later and your friends and family will wish they had done the same as you did. These are the people who are pressuring you, "Come on, you only live once; a little bit won't hurt you." Keep focused on the consequences (future).

Eating When Stressed

When you are stressed, the adrenals overproduce and it becomes difficult to think clearly. You might look for comfort in food. This means you should eat certain things to support your adrenals. These are primarily fats, such as butter, cream cheese, Brie cheese with apples, chicken noodle soup, coconut butter and avocados. These foods greatly stabilize your blood sugar. The worst thing to do is skip a meal and not eat. Hunger is stress to the body. Overeating and stuffing yourself also stress the body. Eating sugar puts stress on the body.

The other thing to do is take calming minerals — potassium, magnesium and calcium. Make sure you do not take the calcium carbonate version, since limestone is not absorbed too well.

When you or your kids consume refined sugar, large quantities of lactic acid build up, which is a byproduct of sugar. Lactic acid makes people restless because it lowers oxygen in the tissues. This is behind restless leg syndrome and hyperactivity in children. Various B vitamins also get depleted when refined sugars and refined grains are eaten. That is why food manufacturing companies enrich grain products with synthetic B vitamins. However, this doesn't work because of the type of vitamin — synthetic made from petroleum material. One of the best sources of B vitamins is nutritional yeast. Put a little in some plain yogurt each day to supply your B vitamins, as lots of mental stress depletes B vitamins.

Also, organize your life so you have healthy foods available. Don't keep sweets at home or at work, since they will always be a temptation. You'll need to purchase some Tupperware and a cooler so you can prepare foods and snacks for the day. Make sure you always have raw nuts, celery, apples, carrots and low-fat yogurt in the cooler as well. By keeping your blood sugars level, it will be easier.

Additional Information on Each Gland

Based on the results of your quiz, along with the other information we have covered, you should now have an idea of what body type you fall into. The following chart will give you additional specifics on each gland.

Vegetables

Liver: Consume lots of cruciferous vegetables, since they support liver function.

Thyroid: Consume lots of noncruciferous vegetables, as cruciferous vegetables tend to deplete iodine (or add some sea kelp, dulse or alfalfa).

Adrenal: Consume lots of vegetables with vitamin C—leafy greens, broccoli, Brussels sprouts, cabbage, cauliflower, bell peppers, parsley, etc.

Ovary: Consume lots of cruciferous vegetables, since they are anti-estrogenic.

Protein

Liver: Start out with small amounts (25 grams) of easily digestible protein (fish, eggs). The liver does not do well on overly cooked or roasted foods.

Thyroid: Consume 25 grams of protein per day. The metabolic rate is slow and it can't tolerate large amounts of protein.

Adrenal: Consume more protein and fat (50–75 grams), as this body type needs to replace the destruction of body proteins (muscles).

Ovary: Consume an adequate amount of protein (50–75 grams) to help trigger fat-burning hormones. Make sure meats are hormone free, since environmental hormones can affect ovaries.

Dietary Fat

Liver: A weak liver can't tolerate fat; consume low-fat foods and use oils sparingly. Coconut oil is the easiest fat to digest and recommended for this type.

Thyroid: The sluggish thyroid can't break down fat properly and many times these people have high cholesterol. Go light on fats.

Adrenal: Adrenal hormones are made from cholesterol. When people experience stress or are sick, their bodies need more cholesterol and fat to build hormones—this is why you might crave fats when you are sick or stressed.

Ovary: The ovarian hormones, like the adrenal hormones, are steroids and are built from cholesterol. This body type can tolerate more fat and cholesterol. Make sure fats are hormone free (butter, cheese, cream, meats and milk).

Minerals

Liver: Since the Liver body type is a fluid-filled belly, which has excess sodium, consuming foods high in potassium is recommended; vegetables, especially cruciferous, have high potassium.

Thyroid: The Thyroid body type needs iodine. However, the diet recommended has enough iodine (in yogurt, eggs, meat, fruits and cheese). If you are concerned, consume sea kelp, dulse or alfalfa.

Adrenal: This body type is losing certain minerals—calcium, potassium and sometimes sodium, depending on what's happening with the adrenals. Consume high-potassium and high-calcium foods—leafy greens are best. If you crave salt, eat some sea salt.

Ovary: The Ovary body type tends to have excessive bleeding during menstruation and the loss of blood depletes iron. Consume red vegetables like beets, red apples and blood-red oranges. The ovaries use iodine like the thyroid does, so it is also a good thing to add sea kelp, dulse or alfalfa to your diet.

Eating Pattern and Frequency

Liver: Because the liver regulates growth hormone and IGF, both of which have a function of controlling blood sugars between meals, it's best to eat three meals but not in between. A good breakfast with protein (as opposed to skipping it) is the most important of all meals.

Thyroid: People with a Thyroid body type crave sugar because of the sluggishness of fuel processing. It is important for these people to eat between meals (protein — raw nuts and seeds) to maintain enough fuel so that blood sugars stay even.

Adrenal: The Adrenal type is dumping lots of stored sugar into the bloodstream or is eating up muscles and turning proteins into sugar. To prevent this, keep protein in the body with small frequent meals — especially between main meals.

Ovary: These people crave chocolate and starches, especially around menstruation. It's vitally important to maintain a protein and fat breakfast mode and to keep sugars low.

Additional Tips

Liver: The Liver type usually has digestive troubles. Consuming fermented foods, such as pickles, sauerkraut, low-fat plain yogurt and low-fat cheese, is recommended.

Thyroid: The thyroid is inhibited by estrogen, so decreasing exposure to estrogen will help this situation — this includes soy products, since soy is estrogenic.

Adrenal: Because the Adrenal type is losing the mineral potassium, the pH of their blood often becomes excessively alkaline. A teaspoon of apple cider vinegar in water before bed is recommended, as this helps stabilize blood pH and potassium (potassium has a relaxing effect).

Ovary: Many times the Ovary body type has ovarian cysts, fibroids, etc. Avoiding estrogenic triggers would be recommended; avoid commercial milks, cheese and meats unless they are hormone free.

Type of Exercise

Liver: To trigger the liver fat-burning hormone (growth hormone), use high-intensity, short-duration exercise (anaerobic). See chapter 14 on this.

Thyroid: Because the thyroid controls the number and size of your mitochondria (cellular energy factories), high-intensity, short-duration exercise is best (anaerobic). See chapter 14 on this.

Adrenal: The adrenal gland is already stressed and exercise will put it into overwhelm. Do light, low-pulse-rate, low-intensity exercise (aerobic). Once the adrenals are stronger, then you can add some anaerobic exercise. See chapter 14 on this.

Ovary: Since most of the fat is superficial and around the legs and buttocks area, walking or biking is best. The Ovary body type should do a combination of both high- and low-intensity exercise. See chapter 14 on this.

12

Liver & Thyroid Meal Plans

The Liver and Thyroid eating plan involves adding more protein (average 25 grams per day) to the Liver Enhancement.

The main differences between Liver and Thyroid meals are

1. Liver eats more cruciferous vegetables and Thyroid consumes noncruciferous vegetables or adds some iodine foods with them (sea kelp, dulse or alfalfa).
2. Liver has no snacks between meals and Thyroid does have snacks between meals.

If you get hungry or are not satisfied, add some more vegetables to these meal plans.

It is also recommended that you keep your omega fats balanced. Most of the nuts and seeds are rich in omega 6; and by adding flax each day, which is high in omega 3 — either 1 teaspoon of flax oil or 3 flaxseed-oil perles — you will maintain the correct ratio of these essential fats.

Food Examples

The following chart gives some examples of quantities of animal proteins per meal. You can use any combination you want as long as the total grams fall within the 25-gram range. This chart doesn't include vegetarian proteins like seeds, nuts and beans, and it is totally okay to exceed the 25-gram daily total with these vegetarian proteins. With the

Liver and Thyroid types, animal proteins need to be on the low side.

These numbers do not have to be exact. If you crave more, go ahead and eat more, as this is a guideline. Some days you might eat 35 grams and other days you might eat 20 grams—don't get hung up on measuring every little thing.

Examples of Liver & Thyroid Animal/Fish/Dairy Protein Amounts per Meal

Breakfast	Lunch	Dinner	Total (per day)
10 g/meal	10 g/meal	5 g/meal	(~25 g)
1 egg (hard-boiled)	1 chicken leg	1 oz cheese	= 24 grams
½ cup cottage cheese	½ cup plain yogurt	No protein	= 26 grams
3 oz steak	No protein	No protein	= 30 grams
No protein	1 chicken breast	No protein	= 20 grams
1 egg	3 oz fish	No protein	= 27 grams
2 oz cheese	½ cup cottage cheese	No protein	= 29 grams
No protein	3 oz hamburger	No protein	= 30 grams
½ cup plain yogurt	½ cup cottage cheese	No protein	= 26 grams
1 chicken leg	2 oz cheese	No protein	= 24 grams

Many people have the idea that 6 oz of meat is 6 oz of protein. However, these are two different things. No food in nature is pure; foods are always combinations of many factors. For example, let's take one egg. It weighs 56 grams yet has only 7–9 grams of protein, 5 grams of fat, 240 mg of cholesterol, and 1 gram of carbohydrate. The rest is a compound of minerals, some fiber, etc. So when we talk about foods that are proteins, we are talking about what they are predominately composed of. Nuts, for example, are fat and protein. Beans are mostly carbohydrate and protein. But as we move away from whole foods and into refined foods, we get more concentrated single categories—table sugar being 100 percent carbohydrate.

Protein Amounts

Amount	Food	Grams of Protein
1	Egg	7 grams
1	Chicken leg	10 grams
1	Chicken breast	20 grams
3 oz	Small can of tuna	20 grams
3 oz	Sardines (in water)	20 grams
6 oz	Large can of tuna	40 grams
3 oz	Fish	20 grams
6 oz	Fish	40 grams
3 oz	Meat/hamburger	30 grams
3 oz	Turkey meat	20 grams
1 oz	Cheese	7 grams
3 oz (½ cup)	Cottage cheese	15 grams
3 oz (½ cup)	Plain yogurt	11 grams
¼ cup	Nuts/seeds	8 grams
2 tbsp	Peanut butter	9 grams
1 cup	Beans	15 grams

The above chart will give you a quick conversion to grams of different food amounts so that you can combine them to equal roughly 25 grams of animal protein per day. Several vegetarian proteins are listed as well. There is also an illustration of these gram amounts on the next page.

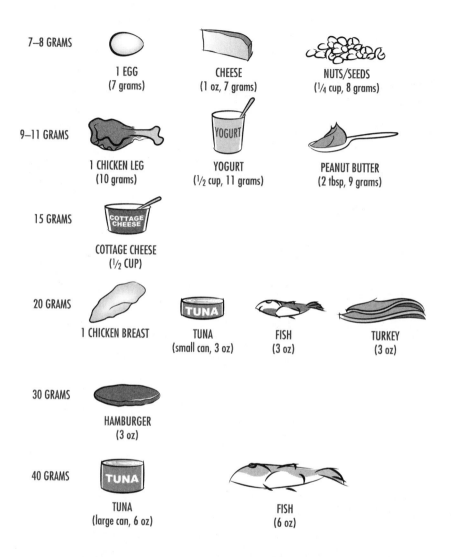

7–8 GRAMS

1 EGG
(7 grams)

CHEESE
(1 oz, 7 grams)

NUTS/SEEDS
(¼ cup, 8 grams)

9–11 GRAMS

1 CHICKEN LEG
(10 grams)

YOGURT
(½ cup, 11 grams)

PEANUT BUTTER
(2 tbsp, 9 grams)

15 GRAMS

COTTAGE CHEESE
(½ CUP)

20 GRAMS

1 CHICKEN BREAST

TUNA
(small can, 3 oz)

FISH
(3 oz)

TURKEY
(3 oz)

30 GRAMS

HAMBURGER
(3 oz)

40 GRAMS

TUNA
(large can, 6 oz)

FISH
(6 oz)

In the following pages I will give you examples of weekly meal plans. Because the Liver type generally needs to have only three meals per day without snacks and the Thyroid type needs food between meals, I have separated the two, with one example for Liver and one for Thyroid.

Example of Weekly Plan for Liver Type

Sunday

Breakfast
- Sautéed mushrooms
- Celery with peanut butter

Lunch
- Chicken breast +
  salad with black olives
  and onions

Dinner
- Green salad (kale) + raw walnuts

Monday

Breakfast
- Tuna with cut vegetables +
  raw walnuts

Lunch
- Plain yogurt + cut vegetables
  (mixed with kale)

Dinner
- Sautéed mushrooms +
  chicken salad

Tuesday

Breakfast
- Eggs
- Apple

Lunch
- 1 cup low-fat cottage cheese +
  baby spinach leaves

Dinner
- Mixed salad + tomatoes

Example of Weekly Plan for Liver Type

Wednesday

Breakfast
- Eggs with cheese chunks + raw almonds and seeds

Lunch
- Cabbage salad with carrots + walnuts

Dinner
- Soup + salad (red cabbage) + sardines

Thursday

Breakfast
- Peanut butter with celery
- Small steak

Lunch
- Steamed beets + green salad with mixed kale

Dinner
- Hard-boiled egg + asparagus topped with butter

Friday

Breakfast
- Low-fat cottage cheese with berries + raw nuts

Lunch
- Steamed collard greens + cheese

Dinner
- Ahi tuna + salad with broccoli

Example of Weekly Plan for Liver Type

Saturday

Breakfast
- Fish
- Asparagus with butter

Lunch
- Cooked Brussels sprouts
  with mixed greens

Dinner
- Broccoli + dip
  (low-fat cheddar cheese)

Example of Weekly Plan for Thyroid Type

Sunday

Breakfast
- Egg omelet with mushrooms
- Bell pepper

Midmorning Snack
- Raw nuts + carrots

Lunch
- Sushi (without rice)
  + romaine salad with feta cheese

Afternoon Snack
- Raw nuts

Dinner
- Low-fat cheddar cheese melted
  over steamed cauliflower

Evening Snack
- Celery

Monday

Breakfast
- Eggs with melted cheese + celery

Midmorning Snack
- Peanut butter on celery

Lunch
- Mixed salad + tomatoes + hot
  chicken wings

Afternoon Snack
- Small apple

Dinner
- Chicken soup + salad (spinach
  leaves and cut pineapple)

Evening Snack
- Orange

Example of Weekly Plan for Thyroid Type

Tuesday

Breakfast
- Egg + cottage cheese and pineapple

Midmorning Snack
- Raw nuts

Lunch
- Fish + green beans slightly steamed

Afternoon Snack
- String cheese

Dinner
- Salad + cheese and kidney beans + raw nuts

Evening Snack
- Apple

Wednesday

Breakfast
- Sautéed mushrooms + turkey slice

Midmorning Snack
- Cheese

Lunch
- Sautéed onions + cut carrots

Afternoon Snack
- Peanut butter on celery

Dinner
- Lentil soup + celery and guacamole dip

Evening Snack
- Raw nuts

Example of Weekly Plan for Thyroid Type

Thursday

Breakfast
- Plain yogurt + raw pecans and pineapple

Midmorning Snack
- Raw nuts

Lunch
- Fish + cucumber and tomatoes

Afternoon Snack
- Carrot sticks

Dinner
- Squash + cut vegetables

Evening Snack
- Berries with yogurt

Friday

Breakfast
- Turkey patty with cut carrots

Midmorning Snack
- String cheese

Lunch
- Egg salad + vegetables (romaine lettuce, avocado)

Afternoon Snack
- Bell pepper sliced

Dinner
- Salad with tomato, cheese, basil + 1 hard-boiled egg

Evening Snack
- Celery

Example of Weekly Plan for Thyroid Type

Saturday

Breakfast
- Roast beef slices with cheese wrapped in lettuce

Midmorning Snack
- Raw nuts

Lunch
- Low-fat cottage cheese with leafy green salad

Afternoon Snack
- Berries

Dinner
- Cut avocado slices, cheese and tomato

Evening Snack
- Apple

Additional Liver & Thyroid Meal Ideas

- Peel, slice and seed an avocado. Fan out on plate; drizzle with extra virgin olive oil and fresh lemon juice. Sprinkle with sea salt.

- Low-fat yogurt with cut fresh pineapple and sliced almonds.

- Top portobello caps with diced fresh tomatoes, diced fresh mozzarella, garlic, basil. Bake until cheese melts.

- Salsa (organic with no sugar added) over scallops.

- Diced tomato, broccoli sprouts and avocado slices. Any vinaigrette. Sea salt to taste. Wrap in Boston or bibb lettuce leaves. (Can add cooked chicken or turkey.)

- Spread apple slices with room-temperature Brie.

- Mixed baby greens topped with sliced beets, walnuts and diced fresh mozzarella, drizzled with balsamic vinaigrette.

- Cucumbers (sliced lengthwise) dipped in guacamole.

- Sliced roasted beets, coarsely broken walnuts, crumbles of feta cheese. Sprinkle with sea salt and pepper. Drizzle with balsamic vinaigrette.

- Spaghetti squash tossed with garlic, butter (or olive oil) and fresh herbs — e.g., parsley, chives, oregano.

- Low-fat yogurt with puréed strawberries.

- Brie cheese with cut pears and walnuts.

- Chopped tomatoes, chopped green onion, shredded carrot, broccoli sprouts and hummus. Wrap in Boston or bibb lettuce leaves.

- Hummus with chopped kalamata olives and celery sticks.

- Cucumber slices dipped in baba ganoush.

- Feta cheese chunks with black or green olives, tomatoes and garlic.

See chapter 10, page 163, for further examples of Quick Healthy Small Meals & Snacks.

A Few of Dr. Berg's Favorite Recipes for the Liver & Thyroid Plan

SUGAR SNAP PEAS WITH LEMON MUSTARD DRESSING

1 lb sugar snap peas cut diagonally into ¼-inch slices

Juice from 1 medium lemon

1 tbsp Dijon-style mustard

6 drops clear stevia

5 tbsp olive oil

¼ cup Canadian bacon julienned (unprocessed and organic)

2 tbsp green onions, finely minced

Sea salt

Bring a pot of salted water to a boil. Add the peas to the boiling water and cook until almost tender but still a little crisp, approx. 3 minutes. Plunge the peas into a bowl of ice water to stop them from cooking further and drain.

Whisk together the lemon juice, mustard, stevia and olive oil; add salt to taste.

In a large bowl, gently toss together the peas, Canadian bacon, green onions and dressing.

Serve at room temperature.

A Few of Dr. Berg's Favorite Recipes for the Liver & Thyroid Plan

SPAGHETTI SQUASH WITH TAHINI

1 medium spaghetti squash

4 tbsp tahini

1 tsp finely minced garlic

1 tbsp lemon juice

⅓ cup chicken stock

2 tbsp chopped chives

Sea salt

Roast the squash at 350 degrees until the shell can be pierced easily with a fork.

Cut the squash in half lengthwise and scoop out seeds. With a fork gently scrape out the flesh in strands to resemble spaghetti. Keep squash warm.

Bring stock to a simmer and stir in tahini, garlic and lemon juice. Toss the squash with the tahini mixture and chives, and salt to taste.

A Few of Dr. Berg's Favorite Recipes for the Liver & Thyroid Plan

ASPARAGUS AND TOMATO FRITTATA

2 eggs

½ cup asparagus, sliced diagonally into 1-inch pieces

1 medium plum tomato diced (approx. ½ cup)

4 tbsp yogurt

Sea salt, to taste

1 tbsp butter

Preheat broiler.

Beat eggs in a small bowl with yogurt and salt. Yogurt blends more easily if stirred until smooth before adding to eggs.

Preheat 8-inch frying pan over medium heat. When pan is hot but not smoking, melt butter. Cook asparagus until just tender, approx. 3 minutes. Add eggs and tomatoes to the pan and stir with a fork until just blended. Allow eggs to set on the bottom for 1 to 1½ minutes. Remove the pan from heat and slip under the broiler until the top of the frittata is just set and puffy. Watch closely; this will only take about a minute. Serve immediately.

A Few of Dr. Berg's Favorite Recipes for the Liver & Thyroid Plan

---

SESAME GINGER KALE SLAW

Dressing

⅓ cup rice vinegar

2 tbsp soy sauce

1 tbsp Dijon mustard

1 tbsp raw honey

1 tbsp chopped garlic

2 tbsp minced or grated ginger

Sea salt, to taste

¼ cup sesame oil

¼ cup safflower oil

2 tbsp sesame seeds

In a blender, combine the first seven ingredients. While blender is running, drizzle in the oils and blend well. Stir in sesame seeds. Refrigerate until chilled. Lightly dress shredded or finely chopped kale, shredded carrots, thinly sliced red onion and chopped walnuts (if desired). Toss well before serving.

A Few of Dr. Berg's Favorite Recipes for the Liver & Thyroid Plan

KALE SLAW

Dressing

1 egg

1 tbsp raw honey

2 tsp celery seed

1 tsp dry mustard

½ tsp sea salt

½ cup cider vinegar

1½ cups safflower oil

In a blender, combine all ingredients except oil. While blending on high speed, slowly drizzle in the oil. Refrigerate.

Just before serving, lightly dress shredded or finely chopped kale, shredded carrots and thinly sliced red onion. Toss well and serve.

13

Adrenal & Ovary Meal Plans

The eating plan for the Adrenal and Ovary types includes more protein, fats and oils than for the Liver and Thyroid plan. I have found, generally speaking, that Adrenal and Ovary types do not do well on just vegetables, as with the Liver Enhancement. They either feel fatigued and lethargic without enough protein or they feel bloated on lots of vegetables. They do much better on the following meal plans.

With the extra protein, it is important to consume grass-fed animal products as well as wild-caught fish. Also, add 1 teaspoon of flax oil or 3 flaxseed-oil perles per day to the plan, as this will supply the necessary omega 3 fats.

Food Examples

The chart on the next page will give you some quick examples of types of animal protein per meal. You can add additional nonanimal proteins (seeds, nuts, beans, etc.) to this eating plan.

Examples of Adrenal & Ovary Animal/Fish/Dairy Protein Amounts per Meal

Breakfast	Lunch	Dinner	Total (per day)
20–30 g/meal	20–30 g/meal	10–15 g/meal	~50–75 g
3 eggs (hard-boiled)	1 chicken breast	3 oz cheese	= 62 grams
6 oz tuna	3 oz turkey	1 chicken leg	= 70 grams
6 oz fish	½ cup cottage cheese	No protein	= 55 grams
1 cup cottage cheese	3 oz steak	2 eggs	= 74 grams
3 oz steak	3 oz tuna fish	1 oz cheese	= 57 grams
3 oz hamburger patty	3 oz fish	1 egg	= 57 grams
3 oz turkey	5 oz cheese	1 chicken leg	= 65 grams
3 oz cheese	1 chicken breast	½ cup plain yogurt	= 52 grams
½ cup plain yogurt	6 oz tuna	½ cup cottage cheese	= 66 grams

Many people have the idea that 6 oz of meat is 6 oz of protein. However, these are two different things. No food in nature is pure; foods are always combinations of many factors. For example, let's take one egg. It weighs 56 grams yet has only 7–9 grams of protein, 5 grams of fat, 240 mg of cholesterol, and 1 gram of carbohydrate. The rest is a compound of minerals, some fiber, etc. So when we talk about foods that are proteins, we are talking about what they are predominately composed of. Nuts, for example, are fat and protein. Beans are mostly carbohydrate and protein. But as we move away from whole foods and into refined foods, we get more concentrated single categories—table sugar being 100 percent carbohydrate.

Protein Amounts

Amount	Food	Grams of Protein
1	Egg	7 grams
1	Chicken leg	10 grams
1	Chicken breast	20 grams
3 oz	Small can of tuna	20 grams
3 oz	Sardines (in water)	20 grams
6 oz	Large can of tuna	40 grams
3 oz	Fish	20 grams
6 oz	Fish	40 grams
3 oz	Meat/hamburger	30 grams
3 oz	Turkey meat	20 grams
1 oz	Cheese	7 grams
3 oz (½ cup)	Cottage cheese	15 grams
3 oz (½ cup)	Plain yogurt	11 grams
¼ cup	Nuts/seeds	8 grams
2 tbsp	Peanut butter	9 grams
1 cup	Beans	15 grams

I've given you this chart again, along with the illustration of grams on the following page, to use in determining your protein amounts. These will fluctuate more or less, depending on individual body size. If you are a large individual and crave more protein, add more; however, animal proteins should stay within the 50- to 75-gram daily total.

The amount of protein you need in this range depends on how much you weigh. If you weigh more than 200 pounds, the protein amount will be on the high side (75 grams per day). If your weight is 180 pounds or less, your proteins will need to be on the low side (50 grams per day). If you are between 180 and 200 pounds, the amount should be somewhere in between. However, I do not want you to get hung up on exact grams. Just consume what feels satisfying to you.

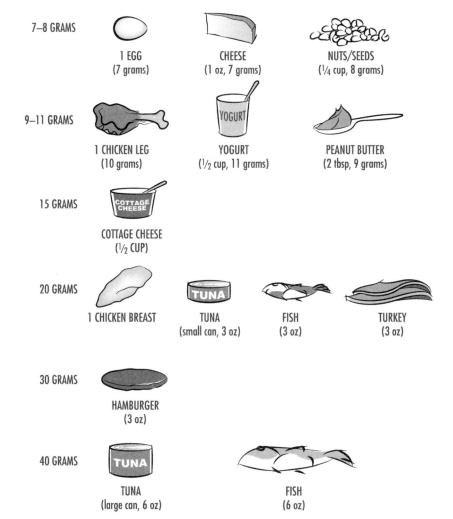

7–8 GRAMS

1 EGG
(7 grams)

CHEESE
(1 oz, 7 grams)

NUTS/SEEDS
(¼ cup, 8 grams)

9–11 GRAMS

1 CHICKEN LEG
(10 grams)

YOGURT
(½ cup, 11 grams)

PEANUT BUTTER
(2 tbsp, 9 grams)

15 GRAMS

COTTAGE CHEESE
(½ CUP)

20 GRAMS

1 CHICKEN BREAST

TUNA
(small can, 3 oz)

FISH
(3 oz)

TURKEY
(3 oz)

30 GRAMS

HAMBURGER
(3 oz)

40 GRAMS

TUNA
(large can, 6 oz)

FISH
(6 oz)

Example #1 of Weekly Plan for Adrenal & Ovary Types

Sunday

Breakfast
- Egg omelet with mushrooms
- Raw nuts

Midmorning Snack
- Cheese + carrots

Lunch
- Tuna salad + raw nuts

Afternoon Snack
- Hard-boiled egg

Dinner
- Salmon + cooked
  Brussels sprouts

Evening Snack
- Celery

Monday

Breakfast
- Turkey bacon + eggs with
  melted cheese

Midmorning Snack
- Nothing

Lunch
- Hamburger patty + cut vegetables

Afternoon Snack
- Celery + peanut butter

Dinner
- Chicken + pineapple and lettuce

Evening Snack
- Celery

Example #1 of Weekly Plan for Adrenal & Ovary Types

Tuesday

Breakfast
- Eggs
- Sautéed mushrooms

Midmorning Snack
- Raw nuts

Lunch
- Steak + salad (red cabbage)

Afternoon Snack
- Raw nuts + cheese

Dinner
- 3 oz roast beef +
  cheese and celery

Evening Snack
- Berries

Wednesday

Breakfast
- Plain yogurt with berries
  and raw nuts

Midmorning Snack
- Cheese + carrots

Lunch
- Roast beef wrapped in lettuce

Afternoon Snack
- Nothing

Dinner
- 6 oz London broil
  + veggies

Evening Snack
- Celery

Example #1 of Weekly Plan for Adrenal & Ovary Types

Thursday

Breakfast
- Steak and eggs

Midmorning Snack
- Nothing

Lunch
- Melted cheese over chicken patty + broccoli chunks

Afternoon Snack
- Hard-boiled egg

Dinner
- Soup + salad (kale) + raw walnuts

Evening Snack
- Brie cheese melted over apples and raw pecans

Friday

Breakfast
- Turkey patty with cheese

Midmorning Snack
- String cheese

Lunch
- Chicken breast + salad

Afternoon Snack
- Peanuts

Dinner
- Kidney beans + roast beef

Evening Snack
- Apple

Example #1 of Weekly Plan for Adrenal & Ovary Types

Saturday

Breakfast
- Eggs hard-boiled
- Chicken leg

Midmorning Snack
- Nothing

Lunch
- Turkey + sauerkraut

Afternoon Snack
- Apple

Dinner
- Fish + coleslaw

Evening Snack
- Pineapple chunks

Example #2 of Weekly Plan for Adrenal & Ovary Types

Sunday

Breakfast
- Egg omelet with avocado slices + raw spinach

Midmorning Snack
- ½ cup plain yogurt

Lunch
- Tuna + salad

Afternoon Snack
- Raw nuts + carrots

Dinner
- Cheddar cheese broccoli + 3 oz turkey

Evening Snack
- Nothing

Monday

Breakfast
- Eggs with melted cheese
- Yogurt

Midmorning Snack
- Peanut butter on celery

Lunch
- Chicken breast + vegetables (kale)

Afternoon Snack
- Nothing

Dinner
- Soup and salad + 3 oz lamb

Evening Snack
- Apple

Example #2 of Weekly Plan for Adrenal & Ovary Types

Tuesday

Breakfast
• Steak + eggs

Midmorning Snack
• Raw nuts

Lunch
• Beef + cheese rolled up in lettuce

Afternoon Snack
• Cheese sticks

Dinner
• Salad + 3 oz fish

Evening Snack
• Raw nuts

Wednesday

Breakfast
• Yogurt and berries

Midmorning Snack
• Cheese

Lunch
• Turkey + salad

Afternoon Snack
• Peanut butter on celery

Dinner
• Seafood stew + sauerkraut

Evening Snack
• Nothing

Example #2 of Weekly Plan for Adrenal & Ovary Types

Thursday

Breakfast
- Chicken + cheese

Midmorning Snack
- Raw nuts

Lunch
- Fish + vegetables

Afternoon Snack
- Raw nuts

Dinner
- Soup + cut vegetables
- 1 cup of cottage cheese

Evening Snack
- Orange

Friday

Breakfast
- Hamburger patty with cheese

Midmorning Snack
- String cheese

Lunch
- Hard-boiled eggs + vegetables

Afternoon Snack
- Vegetable sticks
  (carrots and bell peppers)

Dinner
- Salad with grilled chicken

Evening Snack
- Nothing

Example #2 of Weekly Plan for Adrenal & Ovary Types

Saturday

Breakfast
- Hard-boiled eggs
- Grilled onions

Midmorning Snack
- Raw nuts

Lunch
- Steak patty + salad

Afternoon Snack
- Nothing

Dinner
- Chicken skewers +
  cut vegetables

Evening Snack
- Raw nuts

Eggs — the Almost Perfect Food

The egg is nearly the perfect food for health and weight loss. It is easily digestible as well as a complete food. Eggs give the liver the building blocks it needs to regenerate. Cholesterol levels are not increased by eating them and you can lose weight by including them in your diet. The only time I would avoid eggs is if you have a sluggish or no gallbladder.

Eggs contain ingredients to develop a healthy body including nearly all of the essential nutrients, such as B_1, B_6, folic acid and B_{12}. They contain the key minerals calcium, magnesium, potassium, zinc and iron. Choline and biotin, which are important for energy and stress reduction, are also found in eggs, and they are complete in all amino acids (protein building blocks).

The fats in the egg yolk are in nearly perfect balance. These essential fats are crucial in the regulation of cholesterol. That is because the antidote to cholesterol is lecithin, which helps dissolve cholesterol, and egg yolks are loaded with lecithin. Make sure not to overcook the yolks, as this will destroy the lecithin. These yolk fats in your diet lower the risk of heart disease. Eggs have almost zero carbohydrates and have the highest rating for complete proteins (containing all the amino acids) of any food. Amino acids are necessary for repairing tissue as well as for making hormones and brain chemicals.

As a side note, many people are afraid of eating egg yolks because of cholesterol. The fact is that most of the cholesterol in our blood is there not because of what we've eaten. Actually, our livers make approximately 75 percent of the cholesterol that exists in our blood. The more cholesterol we eat, the less the body will make. The less cholesterol we eat, the more the body will make. If cholesterol were so bad for us, why would our bodies make so much? The body is an incredible system that knows exactly what to do to create synergy. When we consume foods containing cholesterol, we only absorb 2 to 4 mg of cholesterol per kilogram of body weight per day. So, even if we were to eat a dozen eggs each day, we would only absorb 300 mg, which is, by the way, the recommended maximum daily amount.

Omelet Ideas

Mix 2 to 3 eggs with sea salt and 2 tbsp of cream until fluffy. Melt ⅛ stick of butter in a pan over medium heat; pour eggs in pan and lightly cook for 1 minute. Place mixture of fillings on top and flip one side of omelet over until the omelet is slightly browned.

Omelet Chart

- eggs + goat cheese
- eggs + salsa
- eggs + sautéed mushrooms and onions
- eggs + ground turkey and cheese
- eggs + red peppers and spinach
- eggs + cut tomatoes and green peppers
- eggs + crab and cheese
- eggs + 3 cheeses
- eggs + chicken chunks and cheese
- eggs + avocado slices
- eggs + cream cheese
- eggs + cheese and broccoli
- eggs + meatballs and tomato sauce
- eggs + salmon and cheddar cheese
- eggs + basil leaves and melted cheddar cheese
- eggs + ground beef and Parmesan cheese
- eggs + sun-dried tomatoes with onions and basil leaves
- eggs + tomatoes, mushrooms and onions
- eggs + zucchini and eggplant

A Few of Dr. Berg's Favorite Recipes
for the Adrenal & Ovary Plan

CURRIED CHICKEN SALAD

4 cups poached chicken, cut in chunks

3 cups sliced celery

2 cups chopped apples

1 cup fresh pineapple

½ tsp sea salt

½ cup sliced almonds

2 tbsp lemon juice

Curry mayo (see recipe on next page)

Combine all ingredients. Chill.

222 | The 7 Principles of Fat Burning

A Few of Dr. Berg's Favorite Recipes
for the Adrenal & Ovary Plan

Curry Mayonnaise

  1 large egg

  1 tbsp good curry powder

  ½ tsp sea salt

  ¼ tsp freshly ground white pepper

  1 tbsp lemon juice

  1 cup safflower oil

Place everything but the oil in a blender or food processor container. Process 5 seconds in the blender, 15 seconds in the processor. With the motor running, add the oil, first in a drizzle, then in a thin, steady stream. When all the oil has been added, stop the motor and test for consistency. If the sauce is too thick, thin with a small amount of hot water or lemon juice. If too thin, process a little longer.

A Few of Dr. Berg's Favorite Recipes for the Adrenal & Ovary Plan

WALNUT CHICKEN

1½ cups walnuts

5 cloves garlic, roughly chopped

¾ cup boiling water

2 tsp red wine vinegar

½ tsp sea salt

1 tsp crumbled saffron threads

¾ tsp ground coriander

¼ tsp paprika (preferably Hungarian)

Dash cayenne pepper

6 boneless, skinless chicken breasts

For the sauce:

Early in the day, pulse the nuts coarsely in a food processor. Add the garlic and continue to pulse until the mixture is a paste. Transfer to a bowl and gradually stir in the boiling water, stirring constantly until smooth. Stir in the vinegar and spices. Allow to stand several hours for the flavors to blend. Do not refrigerate.

When ready to cook chicken, preheat oven to 450 degrees. Rub chicken breasts with a little butter or olive oil and place in a single layer in a shallow pan. Roast for 20 to 25 minutes till there is no pink remaining. Remove from oven and cover loosely with foil. Allow to rest 10 minutes before slicing. Spoon the sauce over the sliced chicken and serve.

A Few of Dr. Berg's Favorite Recipes
for the Adrenal & Ovary Plan

GARLIC WALNUT CHICKEN

4 bone-in chicken breast halves

Sea salt

Freshly ground black pepper

2 tbsp butter

1 tbsp safflower oil

10–12 cloves garlic, peeled

1 cup walnuts

1 cup water

Season the chicken with salt and pepper.

In a large skillet, heat the butter and oil. Sauté chicken on each side over medium heat for 3 to 4 minutes. Cover the pan and continue to cook until the chicken is done.

Meanwhile, in the food processor, grind the walnuts and garlic until fine, but not a paste.

When chicken is done, remove from pan and keep warm. Drain the pan, reserving 4 tbsp of the drippings. Add the ground garlic and nuts to the pan and sauté on medium heat for 2 minutes. Add the water and simmer for 5 more minutes. Return the chicken to the pan, turning it to coat with the sauce. Heat through before serving.

A Few of Dr. Berg's Favorite Recipes for the Adrenal & Ovary Plan

CHICKEN WITH ASPARAGUS

4 boneless, skinless chicken breast halves

2 tbsp olive oil

1 tsp ground coriander

Sea salt and freshly ground pepper

20 asparagus spears

1 cup chicken stock

1 tbsp lemon juice

1 tbsp cold butter

1 tbsp chopped parsley

Slice chicken into ¼-inch strips. Sprinkle the chicken strips with salt, pepper and coriander. Heat the oil in a heavy skillet and sauté the chicken in batches for 3 to 4 minutes until lightly browned and all the chicken is cooked. Keep chicken warm. Add the stock and asparagus to the pan and simmer 4 to 5 minutes until the asparagus is nearly tender. Remove from pan and keep warm with chicken. Add lemon juice to juices in pan and swirl in butter to thicken. Pour over chicken and asparagus and sprinkle with parsley.

A Few of Dr. Berg's Favorite Recipes for the Adrenal & Ovary Plan

CHICKEN PAPRIKASH

4 boneless, skinless chicken breasts cut in large pieces

2 tbsp safflower oil

1 medium onion, finely chopped

1 tsp Hungarian paprika

1 yellow pepper, halved and sliced

1 tomato, halved and sliced

Sea salt, to taste

½ cup yogurt

2 tbsp chopped parsley (optional)

Sauté the onion in oil over medium heat until golden. Remove from heat and sprinkle with paprika. Stir in pepper, tomato, chicken and salt. Cover and cook gently over medium-low heat until chicken is just done. Remove from heat, stir in yogurt and serve with a sprinkle of parsley.

A Few of Dr. Berg's Favorite Recipes for the Adrenal & Ovary Plan

WARM CHICKEN SALAD

4 boneless, skinless chicken breasts

½ lb snow peas

6 cups mixed lettuce, washed and dried

3 carrots, peeled and cut into julienne pieces

2 cups sliced button mushrooms

1 tbsp chopped cilantro

Dressing/Marinade

½ cup lemon juice

2 tbsp whole-grain mustard

1 cup olive oil

4 tbsp sesame oil

1 tsp ground coriander

Mix all dressing ingredients together. Place chicken in a shallow container with half the dressing. Cover tightly and refrigerate 8 hours or overnight. Store the remaining dressing in the refrigerator.

Assembling the salad:

Broil the chicken until cooked through. Allow to rest 10 minutes.

Cook the snow peas in boiling water for 2 minutes, drain and run under cold water to stop cooking process.

Tear the lettuce into bite-sized pieces and combine with the other vegetables in a serving bowl. Slice the chicken thinly and distribute over the salad. Toss with dressing and sprinkle with chopped cilantro.

A Few of Dr. Berg's Favorite Recipes for the Adrenal & Ovary Plan

---

CHICKEN WITH HERBED CHEESE

4 boneless, skinless chicken breast halves

½ cup low-fat ricotta cheese

1 egg, beaten

2 tbsp minced parsley and chives or other herbs as desired

1 tsp crushed garlic

1 tsp minced onion

3 tbsp melted butter

Sea salt

Freshly ground pepper

Preheat oven to 450 degrees.

With a sharp knife, cut a pocket in each chicken breast.

In a small bowl, combine the cheese with the egg and mix thoroughly. Stir in the herbs, garlic and onion.

Using a small spoon, stuff each breast with several tablespoons of the cheese mixture. Fasten with toothpicks if necessary. Season both sides with salt and pepper and arrange in a single layer in an oiled shallow roasting pan. Pour melted butter over the breasts.

Bake for approximately 25 minutes or until chicken is no longer pink. Turn once when halfway done to brown both sides. Let chicken rest 5 minutes before serving.

A Few of Dr. Berg's Favorite Recipes for the Adrenal & Ovary Plan

EASY MEATLOAF

2 lbs extra lean ground beef

6–8 oz portobello mushroom caps

2 eggs

½ cup medium hot salsa*

1½ tsp sea salt

1 tsp pepper

Preheat oven to 375 degrees.

Mince mushroom caps in a food processor until very fine.

In a large bowl, stir together minced mushrooms, eggs, salsa, salt and pepper.

If salsa is chunky, break up large pieces.

Using your hands, thoroughly mix ground beef with mushroom mixture.

In a shallow baking dish, form meat mixture into a loaf. Bake for 1 hour or until internal temperature reaches 160 degrees.

---

*   Picante sauce or *pico de gallo* can be substituted.

14

Exercising for Your Body Type

Exercising but Still Can't Lose?

You would be shocked to find out how little is known about exercise when it comes to triggering fat-burning hormones. In this chapter, you'll learn the essentials of using exercise as a tool to influence maximum fat burning. You will also discover a new approach that is designed to *burn the most fat* during exercise for your body type and why using the wrong kind of exercise can actually stop weight loss.

There are two principal kinds of exercise: (1) low-intensity, low-pulse-rate endurance exercise, called *aerobic*; (2) higher-intensity, higher-pulse-rate resistance exercise, called *anaerobic*.

If you have an Adrenal body type, you will start with aerobic exercise, because the adrenals are already overworked and putting them into too much stress would make things worse. Overstimulating the adrenals can trigger the stress hormone cortisol, and cortisol can make you fat. With Adrenal types, intense exercise will block the rejuvenation and repair of the body. In some cases, the person will even gain weight with exercise.

Some people with large bellies think they need to just work their abs and the weight will melt off because the abdominal muscles are in the same location as this fat, but that is not how it works. This belly fat is not coming from a lack of exercising of the abdominal muscles; it is coming from the hormone cortisol.

The Ovary body type is a lower-body cellulite fat, which needs a combination of endurance and resistance exercise. Liver and Thyroid body types, on the other hand, respond best to anaerobic (intense) exercise.

However, if you are fatigued, I don't recommend you even start exercising. Let the eating plan build up your energy, and then add in exercise.

Athletes in training, on the other hand, are in a completely different situation and may actually want to train using both aerobic and anaerobic exercise. And for many young people and those who still have their full metabolic systems intact, weight loss may come easily from using either method.

Exercise Doesn't Burn Fat: It Triggers Fat-Burning Hormones to Burn Fat

Exercise is just one of many triggers for fat-burning hormones.

Exercise *n.* a regular series of specific movements designed to stress and activate muscles, causing new cellular adaptations and developments— not merely the burning of calories.

According to this definition, you have to be willing to stress your muscles, which can be uncomfortable.

With a healthy body, the body will very quickly adapt to the stress of exercise, increasing its ability to handle more stress. This is why you have to keep raising the level of difficulty and adding stress in order to continue burning fat.

These physical stresses activate hormones that rebuild and make the body's tissues more able to adapt to new stresses. This requires changes in cellular structures—new enzymes, new capillaries, new mitochondria and larger muscle fibers; and when the body is rebuilding during the rest phase (down time), it uses fat as energy to allow this to occur.

The problem lies with the body's dislike of stress; it has a tendency to want to avoid stress—especially the stress of exercise, since it is uncomfortable pushing through the phases of adaptation. However, to stay in fat burning, you have to continue to make exercise uncomfortable. As soon as you become accustomed to the routine, fat burning stops because the hormones have adapted.

Basic Principles of
Exercise and Hormones

There are two basic ways a person could exercise and many variations in between. You could keep the intensity low and exercise for a long time; you could also increase the intensity and exercise for very little time. Each action affects hormones differently.

From a hormone point of view, to create the maximum fat burning you would be better off exercising at high intensity for short time periods with lots of rest in between. This would cause the body to release growth hormone and glucagon,[1] both fat burners. Intense exercise brings about more destruction to the body, influencing hormones to take repair energy from fat. So you are actually destroying the body in order to trigger these hormones to repair and regrow muscle tissue. What's interesting to note is that fat-burning hormones do their work in the rest periods after, *not during*, exercise.

But here's the problem.

If the person is already stressed and their adrenal glands are burnt out, intense exercise can overwhelm the body, creating more damage. This is because of the destructive actions of the hormone cortisol, which tears down muscle tissue, as compared to growth hormone, which builds muscle tissue.

So the Adrenal type's only option is to do low-intensity exercise of longer duration, at least at first. This will cause less stress on the body and it won't take nearly as long to recover. You will trigger some fat burning, but only after 20 to 30 minutes. Most people could even do this daily. However, I would recommend doing it every other day to begin and gradually increasing to daily if possible. This type of exercise is a great way to counter body stress.

Stress in general is regulated by the adrenals. You might have heard about "fight or flight." Well, this is the adrenals' way of reacting to stress. The main hormone triggered is adrenaline; this releases large amounts of stored sugar for quick energy, since the body doesn't have time to burn fat, as it's just too slow. The weaker the adrenals are when going into this program, the less stress you want to experience. Hard-core, intense-type exercise will only irritate the adrenals and release more sugar, not fat. Slow, gentle endurance-type exercise will ease this stress and allow the body to burn more fat and less sugar over time. The goal is to exercise appropriately so as to trigger fat burning and avoid excess stress and sugar burning.

Based on the Body Type Quiz in chapter 4, you will discover what to do first. Those people who have adrenal weakness should start with the low-intensity and then gradually add the higher-intensity exercise.

Calories and Muscle Mass

Calories are units of energy in food.

There is another "popular" idea that building more muscle mass (through anaerobic exercise) will cause the body to burn more calories.

This is absolutely true; *however*, what is the source of those calories being burned? Are they from sugar or fat?

Burning calories by building greater muscle mass does not automatically mean that they will come from *fat* calories. When dealing with weight loss we have to be more concerned with the *type* of calories being burned than with the quantity. When it comes to fat burning, the size of your muscles is insignificant. Look at a football player who has lots of muscle mass yet has lots of fat too. Having large muscles doesn't automatically cause your body to burn more fat.

The most important point to know is that the fat-burning-hormone effect occurs 14 to 48 hours after exercising, BUT only if certain factors are present: adequate sleep, good nutrition, low sugar, low stress and healthy glands.

The following hidden barriers will prevent weight loss:

1. Sleeping less than 7 quality hours. *Quality* means having good deep sleep and feeling rejuvenated.

2. Not resting enough between exercise sessions.

3. Not resting long enough between the repetitions or intense bouts of exercise.

4. Exercising intensely for too long. Intense anaerobic exercise should be kept between 25 and 40 minutes, and even that should include within the workout a good amount of rest between bouts of exercise.

5. Consuming sugars, starches, juice, sports drinks or alcohol. Most protein bars have tons of sugar.

6. Having pain or inflammation.

7. Lots of stress.

Calories Are Insignificant Compared to Hormones

Think about this — if you exercise moderately for 1 hour, you might burn 350 calories. That's equivalent to several teaspoons of salad dressing. No big deal!

The real benefits of exercise occur one to two days later, but *only* if the environment is almost perfect. In other words, if you do things correctly and don't violate the fat-burning environment, you will burn fat. Fat-storing hormones can easily nullify the fat-burning hormones. The worse off your hormone health, the more perfect the other factors need to be.

What you eat before, during and after

Any carbohydrates (except vegetables) will stimulate insulin, which nullifies the fat-burning hormones. This means if you consume sugars 1 hour before or during exercise, you can inhibit the entire purpose of exercise — fat burning. Since fat burning can only occur in the *absence of carbohydrates*, consuming carbs 14 to 48 hours later can also inhibit fat burning. Drinking several alcoholic beverages can set the liver's function back for days, preventing fat burning.

Protein before workouts is best.[2] Eat an egg, some nuts, a small piece of fish or some cheese before exercising.

I had a patient who would reward herself for exercising by going to Dairy Queen every day and wondered why she wasn't losing weight. I had another who would drink half a glass of wine before bed, at the same time working out intensely with no results — I wonder why? Consuming sugar, juice or refined carbohydrates before bed can inhibit fat-burning hormones while you sleep.

The important thing to remember is that a very small amount of carbohydrates through the day can keep you out of fat-burning mode.

Rest between exercises

Rest is crucial between periods of exercise because this is when the body needs energy from the fat to repair itself. You should never exercise over a healing sore muscle. Sore means healing. In most cases, the longer the soreness lasts, the worse off the adrenals. If before the workout you take a teaspoon of flax oil or 3 flaxseed-oil perles (omega 3), this will increase oxygen and speed up the elimination of soreness.

Sleep quality and amount

Insufficient sleep will add stress and keep you from burning fat. One goes through four levels of sleep at night, and it's during deep, rejuvenating sleep that fat-burning hormones take effect, especially within the first few hours. Superficial sleep hinders fat burning.

Stress level

Stress activates cortisol, which has a fat-storing effect. This includes childbirth, divorce, loss of a loved one, pain and inflammation, injury, bad news, work, finances, traffic, and so on.

When losing weight, you should try to maintain a lower stress level. If you find your stress level can't be lowered, you would need to exercise longer — aerobically (light endurance-type).

The Difference between the Body's Two Main Energy Systems

The body, like a machine, needs energy to operate. This requires some type of fuel, in this case food in the form of protein, carbohydrates and fat, which is burned off into energy. You also have stored fuel — sugar and fat.

There are two energy-producing systems in the body that allow us to be in motion. One is for brief high-intensity activity and the other is for low-intensity endurance-type (or long and slow) activity. Under certain circumstances, such as in emergencies or times of sudden intense exertion, we need quick, explosive energy for a short duration. On other occasions, we need longer-lasting endurance-type energy to keep us going for extended periods.

The Aerobic Energy System
Low intensity—longer duration

Aerobic means *with oxygen*. For our purposes here, the aerobic energy system can be defined as burning fuel with oxygen. Your body burns stored fats and stored sugar in the presence of oxygen. An automobile uses a mixture of gasoline and oxygen as its fuel. Similarly, when the body is in the aerobic mode, it uses oxygen in the mixture as well. The aerobic system runs at a turtle's pace—slow to moderate. The heart rate, on average, is between 127 and 130 beats per minute (bpm); however, a better indicator for aerobic exercise is how the person is breathing. A simple way of knowing when you are in the aerobic energy burning state is that you will be able to speak without the need to take gasping breaths during sentences. In other words, you won't be huffing and puffing for air. With this system, *you begin to burn fat after 30 minutes of exercise*, after burning off the body's "limited" sugar supply.

There are several negative things you can do to nullify the benefits of aerobic exercise, as can be seen in the diagram on the next page. The upper line represents the total amount of exercise, while the lighter lower line represents the *actual benefit* after subtracting things like poor sleep, high stress and/or the wrong foods. For example, on Jan. 4 the person worked out for about 100 minutes, but because of what they ate or because they didn't sleep or had too much stress, the actual benefit was zero.

We have created a Web-based Internet tool, called the Fat-Burning-Tracker Coach, which enables you to track these negative factors and ensure you get the maximum fat-burning effects from your exercise time.*

The aerobic energy system is involved in burning fat fuel *during* exercise and slightly after. The other type of exercise, which will be covered in the next section, burns fat *after* bouts of exercise.

---

* For more information, see the resources section, page 313, and Fat-Burning Tracker Web Support, page 331.

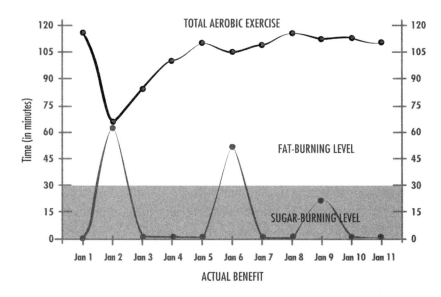

TOTAL AEROBIC EXERCISE MINUS NEGATIVE FACTORS THAT INHIBIT THE BENEFITS OF EXERCISE

Examples of low to moderate activity that would utilize the aerobic energy system include walking, mild treadmill, biking, light jogging, light swimming, light cross-country skiing and other activities where the required heart rate is maintained.

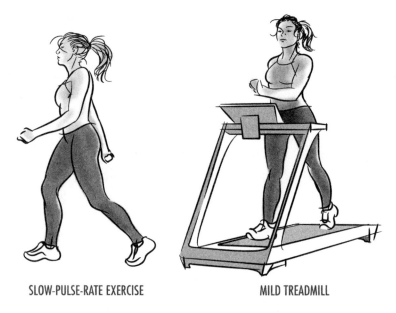

SLOW-PULSE-RATE EXERCISE   MILD TREADMILL

The Anaerobic Energy System
Higher intensity—shorter duration

Anaerobic means *without oxygen*. The anaerobic energy system produces energy without utilizing oxygen; its ONLY source of fuel during the time of exercise is sugar in the blood or stored sugar in the muscles and liver. **This system does NOT initially burn fat fuel during the time you are working out. However, it does stimulate fat-burning hormones 14 to 48 hours later.**[3] (The aerobic system burns fat *during* exercise.) The anaerobic system is used for quick high-intensity exercise and kicks in immediately during exercise when the supply of oxygen becomes inadequate for the activity. Anaerobic gets activated at a higher pulse rate, around 145 beats per minute or greater. It can even get activated with a slow pulse rate if the intensity is high enough.

Some examples of intense exercise that use the anaerobic energy system include running, fast jogging, fast treadmill, soccer, hockey, basketball, swing dancing, wrestling, weight training, sprinting and boxing. It can also include activities such as bike riding and swimming, if the activity is done intensely to the point where the necessary higher heart rate is achieved.

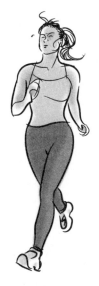

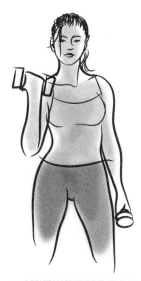

HIGH-PULSE-RATE EXERCISE   **RESISTANCE-TYPE EXERCISE**

Liver/Thyroid Body Type Exercise Plan

Use Anaerobic Only

The fat-burning hormones are stimulated by *intense* exercise. Anaerobic exercise is intense. The more intense it is, the greater the triggering of fat-burning hormones.

The Benefits of Anaerobic Exercise

Even though this system uses *primarily sugar as fuel during exercise (NOT fat)*, it can help stimulate fat burning because of the fat-burning-hormone effects 14 to 48 hours later. It is delayed. But here's the catch — this only occurs if sugar intake and overall stress are low enough and sleep quality and quantity are sufficient. Many people have wasted tremendous amounts of time and energy with very little result simply by not knowing the above facts. They either attempt to use exercise for the wrong body type or self-sabotage by countering the exercise with nullifiers. If you have an Adrenal body type and do intense or high-pulse-rate exercise, you will not usually lose weight.

Another benefit of anaerobic exercise is the triggering of growth hormone. More growth hormone means deeper sleep. Many people get a better quality sleep with anaerobic exercise, as long as they don't work out just before bed.

Growth hormone is the antiaging hormone, and through anaerobic exercise one can keep this hormone within an optimal range. Testosterone also follows growth hormone, which enhances lean muscle mass. Overall, one will burn more fat with anaerobic exercise, but remember there is a day or two delay.

Caution about Anaerobic Exercise

With high-intensity exercise also comes stress. Any stress triggers the hormone cortisol, which can counter the fat-burning hormones. The trick is to exercise intensely enough to trigger fat-burning hormones, yet at the same time keep cortisol (fat-making hormone) low. You accomplish this by SHORT INTENSE BOUTS OF EXERCISE with LOTS OF REST IN BETWEEN. This way the muscles will be activated without stressing the adrenals too much. Overtraining will defeat the entire goal. Once you activate the fat-burning hormones, you can sit back and let them do their job. Make sure you are getting enough rest between exercise periods as well as keeping any and all sugars nil. These are small but important points.

The Hormone Connection to Exercise

To use exercise to trigger fat-burning hormones, it is important to discuss the variables of exercise:

1. Intensity (the power behind the exercise) and difficulty

2. Frequency

3. Duration (total time of exercise)

4. Type

5. Rest

The goal is to use exercise strategically to maximize and keep your body in fat burning and minimize fat-making stress hormones.

Intensity and Difficulty

Intensity is a primary factor; it is the most powerful stimulus for the fat-burning hormones. Growth hormone is the best example of this. If the exercise is not intense enough, you won't be able to stimulate growth hormone.

At the beginning of this exercise program you will stimulate these hormones to burn fat. The body will repair itself and get used to it. The more you get used to the difficulty, the less the fat-burning hormones are affected. So, with time, there will need to be a progressive increase of intensity to create the same effects on fat-burning hormones. You have to keep the difficulty level high in order to keep the intensity high enough. Therefore, you need to keep challenging yourself.

I personally started out biking around my neighborhood on flat pavement. I used to ride my bike through some trails and initially could barely make it up a steep hill—this was intense. Several years later, I am going up very steep hills, which I never thought I could achieve, and it's not even a challenge. So I've had to set my gears lower to make it very difficult going up the hill in order to keep the intensity high. This way I can stay in fat-burning mode. The body adapts and you need to keep challenging it.

Frequency

There are two different frequencies we are talking about. The first is the frequency of repetitions of exercise during one session. The second is how many days per week one exercises.

It is important to keep your workouts short and intense. For anaerobic exercise the repetitions don't have to be many, because as you increase intensity, adding lots of repetitions will also trigger the adrenal stress hormone cortisol and defeat the purpose. If you are doing weight training, instead of increasing repetitions add more weight to increase intensity, but keep the duration short. In the beginning, you'll start out with five repetitions and progress from there. The thing to *not* do is use light weights with a high number of repetitions, as there's not enough intensity to trigger fat-burning hormones.

Anaerobic exercise should be done every other day—not daily—unless you are still sore, in which case you should wait till most of the soreness goes away before working out again. Take more rest between exercises and keep soreness at the low end.

Duration

The actual duration of exercise is also key. If you are being intense and doing it for a long time, you will automatically nullify fat-burning hormones by again stressing the adrenals to pump out cortisol. It's better to keep the intensity high and the duration short and quick. Intense bursts of repetitions for short periods of time, starting at one minute, are best. It is vital to rest for about five minutes between these bouts.*

Types of Exercise

There are two main types of exercise with anaerobic:

1. Weight training or resistance training

2. Increased pulse rate

Since the key to stimulating fat-burning hormones is *intensity*, it is best to find the exercise that will give you the best intensity based on your capabilities. If your body doesn't allow you to do hockey, you might want to stick with either doing weight training or using a resistance machine at the gym, where you could get good intense exercise.

Rest and Recovery

This is the most important variable, as the fat-burning hormones are using up fat during the rest between exercises and up to two days after exercise. Without resting, you get very little fat burning.

With some people, an extra 30 minutes of sleep per night as well as reducing their exercise routine to twice or even once per week, with lots of rest in between, will cause them to start burning more fat.

Plateau

The body adapts to the stress of exercise within two to three weeks. It then takes another two weeks to stabilize these tiny body cell structures. This is why people tend to plateau when attempting to lose weight or when starting any exercise program. This is also why it is crucial to change your exercise routines, keeping them new. I recommend rotating their sequence every two to three weeks. That way your body will never get fully accustomed to the routine and your difficulty and intensity will remain

---

* You can use the Exercise Monitoring Device to help determine your specific recovery rest time. For more information, see the resources section, page 315.

high. This is the most important key to staying in fat burning and getting more out of your exercise. Examples of different types of exercise that can be switched would be biking, step aerobics, running, Curves routines, weight training, yoga, boxing routines, rollerblading, racquetball and swimming. The exception is the Adrenal body type, for which you would want to keep the intensity lower and keep the stress of exercise also on the low side. If you have an Adrenal body type, you would focus on aerobic exercise until your adrenals are stronger, then graduate to higher intensity type exercise.

Hormones Triggered by Anaerobic Exercise

The first one is **growth hormone**. Remember that this is the antiaging, fat-burning, lean-body-mass-producing hormone, which also helps prevent the breakdown of proteins — like your bones, muscles, hair, skin and nails. It is stimulated by intense exercise (anaerobic) only. This hormone works through the liver.

The second one is **glucagon**. This is the opposing hormone to insulin, which gives the cells fuel between meals and is also fat burning. It too works through the liver and is stimulated only by intense exercise.

The third one is **testosterone**. This hormone is made by the adrenal glands, testicles and even the ovaries. It is a fat-burning hormone in that it is involved in making muscle, as well as giving male characteristics and sex drive in males and females. It follows growth hormone — wherever growth hormone goes, so goes testosterone.

The fourth one is **adrenaline**. This is an adrenal hormone and is the main hormone to release fat energy from the fat cells. It is triggered by stress, such as intense exercise.

The above four hormones have something in common — they all work through the liver. In fact, all fat-burning hormones work through the liver. The better the liver works, the better these hormones work. This is why the Liver Enhancement is recommended first. It's interesting that during this period the person is eating mostly vegetables and low amounts of protein, yet their hair, nails and skin are improving. That is because of the liver's increased ability to process more growth hormone, which prevents the breakdown of protein in hair, nails, etc. Now this hormone can help manufacture body proteins more efficiently.

Growth hormone and glucagon are triggered not only by exercise but by consuming dietary protein; however, it has to be the correct amount, as excess protein can turn into fat. The weaker the liver, the less protein the person can handle. So if you fix the liver first, the person can tolerate more protein in the diet and thus get more stimulation of these two fat-burning hormones.

Many people go on a high-protein diet and lose weight for two weeks, then the weight loss stops. This is mainly due to a weakened liver, which cannot break down protein efficiently. They might even show signs of protein deficiency, because the liver is blocking the absorption.

The following chart gives you an idea of when fat-burning hormones are triggered in relation to exercise. The trick is to keep cortisol as low as possible yet at the same time keep the others as high as possible.

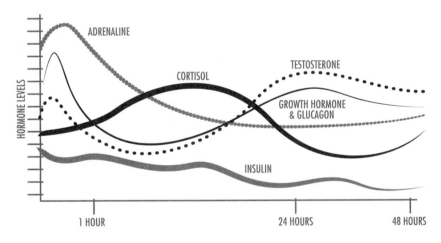

Adapted with permission from Faigin, *Natural Hormonal Enhancement*, 265.

Anaerobic Exercise Routine

1. Keep the intensity high.

2. Do short repetitions of intense exercise, starting at 1 minute.

3. Rest a good amount after each bout of exercise. For example, if you exercise for 1 minute, spend 5 minutes resting afterwards.

4. Exercise between 25 and 40 minutes, but no longer than 45 minutes. This way cortisol will not be raised too high.

5. Exercise every other day with rest between sessions. Do not work out daily.

6. Do not do the entire body; do upper body one day and lower body the next.

7. For the Thyroid type, make sure you only snack on cheese, raw nuts, vegetables or apples before, during and after workouts. If you are a Liver type, eat only three meals per day with no snacking.

8. If your body is sore, wait until the soreness goes away before working out again. It is important that your body heal between sessions, as this means your fat-burning hormones are also working.

Workout example: If you are doing pull-downs on the weight machine, find the weight that is intense enough where you could do 5–7 repetitions. It might take you 30 seconds. Rest for 1 minute. Repeat this 4 times and then rest for 5 minutes. Next, go to bench press and do the same thing. After that, you might want to do rowing, following the same procedure, for 25–40 minutes in all; then you're done.

Workout example: Find how much weight you could squat with, and do 5–7 repetitions. Repeat this 3 times, resting momentarily between reps. After that, rest for 5 minutes. Do the same for hamstrings (back part of the thigh muscle), then leg extensions, for a total of 25–40 minutes.

Workout example: You can do the stationary bike exercise. Get your pulse rate up to 150–180 until your legs fatigue, right around 1–2 minutes. Rest for 5 minutes. Then repeat the same procedure. Do this for a total of 25–40 minutes.

Workout example: Go on a bike ride and get your pulse rate up to 160, then slow down and coast lightly for 5 minutes until your breathing is normal. Do this again and then rest. Repeat this for 25–40 minutes.

Workout example: Do 3–4 sets of push-ups until your arms fatigue, resting a minute between reps. Repeat these 2 additional times with rest in between. Rest for 5 minutes. Then do the same for sit-ups and pull-ups, for a total of 25–40 minutes.

Examples of Anaerobic	Time	Intensity	Difficulty	Soreness
Weight training	25–40 min.	High	Moderate to high	Low
Exercise machine (gym)—resistance	25–40 min.	High	Moderate to high	Low
Home exercise—resistance	25–40 min.	High	Moderate to high	Low
Running	25–40 min.	High	Moderate to high	Low
Sprints	25–40 min.	High	Moderate to high	Low
Sports (basketball, soccer, football, boxing, etc.)	25–40 min.	High	Moderate to high	Low
Biking	25–40 min.	High	Moderate to high	Low
Hiking	25–40 min.	High	Moderate to high	Low
Swing or jazz dancing	25–40 min.	High	Moderate to high	Low
Swimming	25–40 min.	High	Moderate to high	Low
Aerobic dance class	25–40 min.	High	Moderate to high	Low

Anaerobic Exercise Times and Rest Periods

Week	Mon.	Tues.	Wed.	Thurs.	Fri.	Sat./Sun.	Weekly
1	15 min.	REST	15 min.	REST	15 min.	REST	45 min.
2	20 min.	REST	20 min.	REST	20 min.	REST	60 min.
3	30 min.	REST	30 min.	REST	30 min.	REST	90 min.
4	35 min.	REST	35 min.	REST	35 min.	REST	105 min.
5	40 min.	REST	40 min.	REST	40 min.	REST	120 min.
6	40 min.	REST	40 min.	REST	40 min.	REST	120 min.
7	40 min.	REST	40 min.	REST	40 min.	REST	120 min.
8	40 min.	REST	40 min.	REST	40 min.	REST	120 min.

The first chart above shows the factors you should put attention on in anaerobic exercise. The time should be between 25 and 40 minutes, not to exceed 45 minutes. You need enough intense exercise to trigger growth hormone yet not so much that it overstimulates cortisol, which tends to nullify growth hormone. The intensity should be high; on a scale from low to high, you should aim toward high. However, after a while the intensity is relative from person to person, so this needs to continue to increase over time. This also applies to the overall difficulty level (again a relative term from person to person). You should keep it at a moderate to high difficulty level. If it's too easy, fat-burning hormones are not triggered. There is no problem with getting sore after you work out, but you should rest until most of the soreness goes away. In other words, you don't want to exercise over lots of soreness, as you haven't given your body a chance to heal through hormone influences. Also, the adrenal hormone cortisol is activated by soreness and inflammation, so keeping this hormone to a minimum is important.

Keep your anaerobic exercise between 25 and 40 minutes and continue to raise your difficulty level higher over time as your body adapts to the stress you put on it.

The soreness factor is the indicator as to whether or not you should increase the difficulty level. More soreness means hold off and give it more time and more rest. Less soreness means increase the difficulty and intensity.

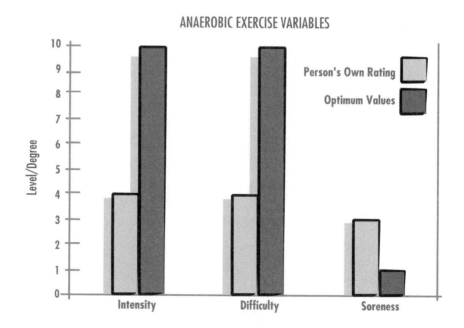

In the following graph, the vertical dark gray bar indicates optimum anaerobic exercise, while the light-colored bar to the right shows the way in which stress, lack of quality sleep and refined carbohydrates nullify exercise. **Our Internet Fat-Burning-Tracker Coach will help you to quickly identify the hidden blockers preventing fat burning.**

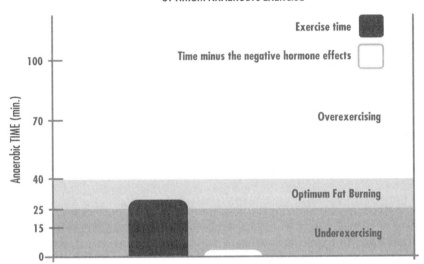

OPTIMUM ANAEROBIC EXERCISE

Adrenal Body Type Exercise Plan

Use Aerobic

If the stress gland is stressed, you want to avoid intense exercise. To improve the stress gland, the correct exercise is calming and less stressful. This type of exercise will burn fat mostly during and slightly after the exercise.

The Benefits of Aerobic Exercise

The main benefit of light endurance-type exercise is that it is very gentle on the adrenals and will keep stress hormones to a minimum. However, aerobic exercise doesn't burn fat 14 to 48 hours after exercise like the anaerobic system does.

The problem with anaerobic exercise is that it can stress the adrenals more than aerobic exercise. More intense exercise and exercise that generates a higher pulse rate triggers the stress part of the nervous system — the "sympathetic nervous system" — which monitors the body's fight-or-flight response. As soon as the body goes into this mode, the stress hormones cortisol and adrenaline kick in. If the adrenals are already overwhelmed, cortisol can become excessive for longer periods of time. This will prevent deep sleep and keep the person in a state of nervous anxiety. Cortisol is also the hormone that produces weight gain in the midsection.

Another positive aspect worth mentioning about the aerobic energy system is that its waste products (carbon dioxide and water) are harmless compared to the waste product from anaerobic exercise (lactic acid). Its only drawback, if you looked hard to find one, is it requires time (at least 20 to 30 minutes of slow exercise with the heart rate between 127 and 130 beats per minute) for the body to even *begin* to burn fat.

Working Harder Will Initially Slow Your Progress

Many people think that to melt a lot of dense fat you need a tremendous amount of intense, hard exercise. This is not true. You can burn fat using only light exercise with little effort. You burn fat while you're barely breathing!

In nearly every patient seminar, I've found that the majority of people who are not losing weight with exercise are mixing weight training into their programs. This is a big mistake if they have an adrenal weakness! Weight training is anaerobic and worsens the adrenal glands.

You can see from the chart on the opposite page the benefits of spending more time doing aerobic exercise. The goal in following this program is to get your body to burn only fat, not sugar. The anaerobic system is working to a small degree during aerobic exercise. But notice what happens to the anaerobic system at 30 minutes; it really shuts down. This is where most people stop exercising — the exact point where the fat burning really begins.

You can also see that if you continue to exercise after the 30-minute point, fat begins to be the predominant fuel; there is great efficiency from this point forward when continuing with aerobic exercise.

Sugar-Burning to Fat-Burning ratios based on time of aerobic exercise

TIME (min.)	% Sugar Burning	% Fat Burning
1	70	30
2	50	50
4	35	65
10	15	85
30	5	95
60	2	98
120	1	99
> 120	< 1	> 99

Aerobic Exercise Routine

1. Keep the intensity low. Keep it light enough so you can breathe comfortably.

2. Start with 15 minutes per day and work up to 60 minutes per day. (Some people will find they can do more than 60 minutes, but the exercise period should be no longer than 120 minutes per day.) Over time you will get used to this and your body will plateau. When that happens, you could add in the anaerobic exercise.

3. Exercise every other day at first with rest in between. After two months, you could progress to daily.

4. Make sure you only snack on cheese, raw nuts, vegetables or apples before, during and after workouts.

5. If your body is sore, wait until the soreness goes away before working out again. It is important that your body heal between sessions, as this means your fat-burning hormones are also working.

With Adrenal types, you have to grow back the muscle you have lost from overactive adrenal glands. Since muscle weighs more than fat, you might not initially lose weight but should feel your clothes getting looser. The weight starts dropping two to three months later in some cases.

Examples of Aerobic	Time
Walking	60 min.
Light jogging	30 min.
Biking	60 min.
Treadmill	60 min.
Elliptical machine	60 min.
Swimming	60 min.
Yoga	60 min.

Aerobic Exercise Times and Rest Periods

Week	Mon.	Tues.	Wed.	Thurs.	Fri.	Sat./Sun.	Weekly
1	15 min.	REST	15 min.	REST	15 min.	REST	45 min.
2	20 min.	REST	20 min.	REST	20 min.	REST	1 hr.
3	30 min.	REST	30 min.	REST	30 min.	REST	90 min.
4	40 min.	REST	40 min.	REST	40 min.	REST	2 hrs.
5	50 min.	REST	50 min.	REST	50 min.	REST	2.5 hrs.
6	60 min.	REST	60 min.	REST	60 min.	REST	3 hrs.
7	60 min.	REST	60 min.	REST	60 min.	REST	3 hrs.
8	60 min.	REST	60 min.	REST	60 min.	REST	3 hrs.

As you can see in the above chart, a gradual progression is best. In the beginning you might not start burning fat because you are working out less than 30 minutes. But it's recommended that you do this, especially if you are not used to it.

If you keep working out for 30 minutes aerobically, you will never burn fat, since fat burning only starts after 30 minutes. It is also recommended that you don't exercise over an hour, since this can stress the adrenals even more. Exercising up to an hour is a safe bet. Once the adrenals are strong, which could take 8 to 12 weeks, you could then add in the anaerobic exercise.

At this point in the program your body will have enough strength to stay in the aerobic mode, and a combination of both types — aerobic and anaerobic — will keep you from adapting to just one form of exercise. As a person gets used to an exercise and it is no longer difficult, fat-burning hormones will cease to be stimulated; so you need to continue varying it and using different muscles, making it more difficult over time.

Don't Stop Before You Start Burning Fat

Based on surveys of people who could not lose weight with exercise, besides those who were mixing anaerobic with aerobic exercise there were many who used only aerobic exercise but they did not do it *long enough* to tap into the fat reserves. In order to get the real benefits of the aerobic energy system, you must exercise long enough — 60 minutes. If you do this, the results will be great.

History of Long-Term Sugar Consumption

If a person has regularly consumed a lot of sugar for some time, it could take even longer to begin burning fat. Even if they were to exercise aerobically, it might take 40 to 50 minutes or more instead of 20 to 30 minutes to start burning fat. This is because their body's sugar reserves have adapted to a larger reserve storage system. You simply need to eliminate sugars completely, and over a few months the body will adapt back to normal sugar supply levels.

Once your body heals, you will be able to add further anaerobic exercise to your program. Anaerobic exercise actually burns more fat than aerobic, but 14 to 48 hours later; yet if your body is in stress mode, it can only tolerate aerobic exercise at first. Using both systems correctly would be the most optimum.

Ovary Body Type Exercise Plan

Use Aerobic and Anaerobic

If you have an Ovary body type, you need to combine BOTH aerobic and anaerobic exercise. You should do this by exercising every day with anaerobic and either every other day or even daily with aerobic.

The type of fat the Ovary body type has is a superficial cellulite. It is mostly below the bellybutton. So the best type of exercise is lower body — walking, running, treadmill, soccer, basketball, jazz dancing, step aerobics, etc. Focus on working the muscles of the hips, thighs and buttocks. Force these muscles to use energy from the surrounding fat layer. The key with the Ovary body type is intensity, really ripping those muscles hard core. This body type needs the most intensity.

Keeping estrogen low is also essential to getting the weight off. This means consuming foods that are antiestrogenic — cruciferous vegetables. It also means avoiding growth hormones (mostly estrogen) in the food supply. I would recommend avoiding soy as well, since soy has plant estrogenic qualities.

Summary

Fat is *potential energy*. Fat has enough potential energy to allow a lean person to run 800 miles or last 90 days without food. But most people, with the exception of long-distance runners, never learn how to tap into this amazing potential. Have you ever noticed that long-distance runners are very thin? This is because they normally remain in the aerobic mode when they run and therefore burn fat as their primary fuel.

Some people (especially Adrenal body types) are initially too unhealthy and fatigued to exercise. If this is the case, we recommend restoring your body's health through correct foods and quality sleep before even starting an exercise program.

15
Questions & Answers

*It seems like my body is a mix of all the types.
Which diet should I use?*

Start with the initial 14-day Liver Enhancement Plan; then, depending on whether you did well or not, add protein as needed. If you did well on the Liver Enhancement, you will continue with this until you crave protein. If something is working, you do not want to change it. In other words, if the Liver Enhancement is working, keep doing it for as long as it continues to work. You could be on this plan for an additional one to three weeks or even up to six months or more.

You will know very early on in the program (even within the first 2 days) if you start to crave protein. Some people have extremely sensitive blood sugar issues and cannot go without protein for very long. Should this occur, you will need to switch to the Liver/Thyroid diet, which includes more protein. On the other hand, if you did not do well on the Liver Enhancement and did not lose weight within the first two weeks, then we'll know you are an Adrenal/Ovary type and need to change to that plan. By not doing well, I mean that you felt fatigued, lethargic, etc.

How much weight loss is possible per week?

There are two types of weight problems: (1) water and (2) fat. The maximum fat that can be burned per week is between one and two pounds. That's it. The maximum water loss is unlimited. This would explain how some people can lose and gain several pounds within days. Anyone can do any diet and lose water weight, but the true test is how much real fat they can lose. This program is designed to directly achieve that. It also emphasizes sodium and potassium food ratios. If you're only losing one to two pounds per week, it might not be a bad thing; it might actually be normal. And it's important to understand this so you don't get discouraged. Better indicators for improvement would be energy level, sleep quality, digestion and cravings, as these tell if the body is healing.

How do I know if I have water weight or fat?

There is a test called Body Composition, which allows a practitioner to measure body fat versus fluids. Generally, if you weigh a lot and get your body fat tested and it comes out low or normal, then you probably have more fluid weight. A fairly large percentage of male patients at my clinic have more water weight than body fat. Exercise rarely fixes this water problem — diet is the only way. Get on the Liver Enhancement Plan to create a healthy liver. Healthy liver foods are high in potassium, which will allow the fluid to come out gradually over a few months. If you notice a very slow, gradual weight reduction, then you know it is fat, not fluid.

What if I do not lose weight?

If a person has major problems with stress, proteins in the muscles (thighs and buttocks) can be broken down and turned into sugar. Sugar is then turned into fat around the abdomen. Some people actually gain weight before they lose weight because the body has to rebuild muscle first, and muscle is heavier than fat. Some of our patients lose inches, increase energy and have better digestion, yet they see no initial weight loss. After these muscles are repaired, I have found that weight loss is easier. Nevertheless, it cannot occur until the body is out of stress mode and in healing mode, and for some people actual weight loss will be delayed for as much as four to eight weeks.

What if I'm pregnant? Can I do this program?

You can follow the meal plans for either Liver & Thyroid or Adrenal & Ovary but not the Liver Enhancement Plan. Just make sure you are adding enough protein. Also, check with your doctor to see if this is acceptable or not. You don't want to be dieting when you are pregnant. However, my program is very healthy and adding proteins to it would help contribute to a healthy baby.

Can I come off my hormone therapy and medications when I'm on this program?

That is between you and your doctor. As you improve, get him or her to help you make the transition.

What if I'm on medication (e.g., Coumadin) that conflicts with consuming certain vegetables?

The medication Coumadin acts like a vitamin K blocker, preventing the clotting of blood. It's used as a blood thinner to prevent clots and strokes. It is also used as a rat poison. Check with your doctor as to what vegetables you can or cannot eat on this program.

Do I have to avoid taking my supplements on this program?

I would recommend that you only avoid them if they are synthetics. Replace them with whole-food-based vitamins.

What vitamins should I take?

I always recommend a food-based vitamin. Look on the back of the label to see if it mentions actual food; then look at the individual ingredients and notice the milligram amounts. If the vitamins are synthetic, you will see the same number of milligrams for each vitamin; for example: 100 mg of B_1, 100 mg of B_2, 100 mg of B_6. The whole-food vitamins come in different amounts; for instance: 21 mg of B_1, 3.4 mg of B_2, or 13 mg of B_6.

Standard Process vitamins are food-based products and, as far as I'm concerned, they are the best available. I have been four times to the farm where they harvest the ingredients and each time I was thoroughly impressed by the quality. To obtain Standard Process supplements, you will need to locate a practitioner in your area who carries them, as they are only sold through healthcare practitioners.*

Your program seems very strict. I'm not sure if I can do it.

Something is better than nothing. Do what you can and try to improve this each week. I had a female patient who just couldn't do the program. However, she was able to do the cranberry drinks and add more vegetables. This helped her to crave less and she was able to do more and more over time. Something is better than nothing.

Do I need to buy all organic, hormone-free foods?

I'm not saying you need to change your entire diet overnight; I'll give you a week. Just kidding. It would be ideal to eat only organic, but 50 percent would be the bare minimum. The first change in your diet needs to be consuming hormone-free foods. Then once this is implemented, start adding the organic (noninsecticide) foods.

I can't afford the organic foods. What should I do?

Get a part-time job to support your new diet. I'm kidding again. You could start with just purchasing organic meats, even hamburger and eggs, and keep everything else commercial. The point? The cost is an investment and it will pay off later. You are basically creating a higher level of health and it's worth the investment. Instead of getting that oil change for your car, buy some organic salad.

---

*   See the entry for Standard Process Inc. on page 315 in the resources section.

The overall protein amounts seem extremely low. Isn't it recommended that a person consume 9 grams per 20 pounds of weight?

Because the cause of stubborn weight is a failing endocrine system, I have found that people can process (digest) less protein than they might have considered. I'm not concerned necessarily about the excess protein adding calories. My concern is that overweight people have poor livers, and too much protein stresses the liver. What benefit is there in adding protein if they are not digesting it? It becomes more of a toxin than a healing food. They actually need more raw whole vegetables. I want them to get their calories from eating lots of vegetables, because it is these vegetables that provide the healing building blocks to repair gland tissue.

How can I be in ketosis when I'm not eating any fat or animal protein?

This is an interesting observation we made. By feeding the body lots of vegetables, very low proteins and no sugars or grains, many people start burning fat and go into ketosis (fat burning). Prove this to yourself: go to the drugstore and purchase some ketone sticks and test your urine in the morning.

Why do I have to do the Liver Enhancement Plan before the diet?

Because ALL fat-burning hormones work through the liver; it is the hub of weight loss.

What if I get constipated on the Liver Enhancement Plan?

If you get constipated on the Liver Enhancement Plan, this means either you are allergic to the vegetables or you are an Adrenal body type. Adrenals do better on more protein. I had one guy get constipated on lots of vegetables and I told him to cut down on them and eat some buffalo burger instead and include other animal proteins with each meal. His bowel movements returned to normal.

For constipation, eat at least half a beet (raw, grated on your salad) daily or drink some prune juice mixed with water—about one-third of a cup in a glass of water. It's sweet, so keep it diluted.

What do I do if I'm allergic to the foods recommended?

Occasionally, a person might think he or she is allergic or has sensitivity to some of the foods recommended, such as broccoli and cabbage. This is more a missing enzyme than an allergy. The person lacks the enzyme needed to digest certain foods, adding stress and bloating to the system and causing gas in the intestines.

I believe this is the result of eating too many cooked and pasteurized foods, which over the years deplete your enzyme reserves. That is why it is important to germinate (soak in water overnight) your seeds and nuts to remove enzyme inhibitors, so that the enzymes in the foods can be reactivated causing less dependency on your own enzyme reserves.

Common gas-producing foods are beans, artichokes, asparagus, broccoli, Brussels sprouts, cabbage, cauliflower, cucumbers, green peppers, onions, radishes, bananas, apricots and pears. Consume vegetables and fruits you know do not cause bloating, as this intestinal stress can increase stress hormones, preventing weight loss.

Make a food log to track your responses and start replacing foods that you are sensitive to with foods you know you can eat without the bloating. Many people are sensitive to cashew nuts, which make them feel bloated and tired. I think this is because most cashews one buys are cooked or roasted, which puts more strain on the body's enzyme reserves. If you experience bloating with any foods, either germinate them (if nuts or seeds) or avoid them, or you can add the missing enzyme to digest these foods—go to http://www.bean-zyme.com/.

What if I just don't like vegetables or can't get enough in my diet?

It is highly recommended that you consume as many vegetables as you can. However, there is something you could do to make up for the lack of quantity. You could consume better quality nutrition, like sprouts. A small serving of sprouts gives you just as much nutrition as a larger quantity of mature vegetables. So you wouldn't be eating as much, just a better quality to get the same nutrition. Eat a small bowl of sprouts with salad dressing or put them in a sandwich.

I can't stand the thought of consuming vegetables for breakfast on the Liver Enhancement. What are the substitutes?

Consume an apple and some nuts. Have cottage cheese or plain yogurt with berries. You could make a shake with berries, plain yogurt and peanut butter. Also, take some celery and dip it into peanut butter or hummus. Apples and hummus are good as well. However, if anytime within three days you don't feel right, add fish for breakfast.

Can't I eat some oatmeal for breakfast?

Preferably not—not until the Maintenance Plan. If you eat it once in a while, it's not a problem, but definitely not on the Liver Enhancement Plan. If you consume oatmeal, make sure it's steel cut, from a health food store.

I'm not hungry for breakfast. Is it okay to skip it?

No, because you will trigger cortisol and crave sweets later at night. You have to eat something, even if it's small, preferably six times per day. If you definitely have a Liver body type, eat only three meals per day with no snacks.

The Liver Enhancement is very low in protein. While I'm on this plan, how do I know when I need to start introducing protein into the diet?

Indications could include cravings for protein or feeling tired, dizzy, lightheaded, extra cold, or like your blood sugars are low. Just start increasing proteins by 10 grams per day to see if this is the reason. And by the way, the absolute best high-quality complete protein you can eat is the egg.

But you have to realize that when you come off coffee for these two weeks—if you do it too quickly—there will be a one- to two-day period of lethargy or grogginess. Just persist and push through this period.

I thought eggs were bad for me and would give me high cholesterol.

Eggs will not increase cholesterol because they are loaded with the antidote—lecithin. I've been eating eggs for the past 17 years without any problem whatsoever, and my cholesterol levels have been below 200 for years.

The only time I would recommend replacing eggs with fish would be if you have a gallbladder problem. And even then, a small number of eggs in the diet would not be much of an issue.

Should I consume just the egg white and skip the yolk?

Eat the whole thing. You need this cholesterol to help with building hormones, especially the adrenal hormones. And the more stress you go through, the more fatty foods, especially eggs, I would recommend. Cholesterol also helps in supporting normal nerve and brain function.

Can I eat eggs daily without a problem?

Yes.

Why can't I have protein powders?

They are too processed (broken down). You need to eat real whole, mostly raw food. There is one exception, however—a product called SP Complete from Standard Process. This is a whey and brown rice protein powder, which is of very high quality.

What is the best thing for brain fog or fatigue around my eyes?

You need more protein for breakfast. This is the most important meal of the day and adding protein (fish, eggs, etc.) is essential to keep your blood sugars level through the day. A lean steak for breakfast is also acceptable. Your stomach is able to digest animal proteins better in the a.m. than the p.m. We recommend that, if possible, a person go without animal protein for the first two weeks.

I'm getting a cold sore (virus) outbreak on the Liver Enhancement. What should I do?

Certain nuts, especially peanuts, and vegetables (except avocados) are higher in an amino acid called arginine as compared with lysine. The amino acid arginine tends to allow viruses to come out of remission creating outbreaks, while lysine does the opposite. Lysine fights cold sores and herpes virus infections. Foods high in lysine are cottage cheese, wheat germ, eggs and chicken. The adrenal glands also closely regulate the immune system in regard to resistance to viruses and infection. Getting cold sores could mean you are more of an Adrenal type, which requires more protein (especially animal protein).

What can I do for itching around different parts of my body, including the soles of my feet?

Itching can be a sign of liver issues. When the liver can no longer break down histamines, you experience itching. I recommend taking two amino acids—one called glycine and the other, taurine. These both improve liver function.

I'm bored with the food and need something to snack on other than apples, nuts and vegetables. What can I do?

Thin Rye Crisp crackers are better than wheat crackers, and dipping them into some Brie cheese would be okay. You could also dip them in hummus, salsa or melted cheese. Bran Crispbread is another idea; these crackers are very low in carbohydrate and high in fiber.

Or you could have melted Brie cheese with pecans. Put it in the oven with the nuts and it makes a great snack or meal. Use an apple to dip into the mixture.

A further suggestion is Greek yogurt (plain) with some walnuts and a very small amount of honey. Use Tupelo or raw honey. It's interesting to note that the bees around some Tupelo trees make 30,000 trips to the beehives to create one pound of honey. It is one of the slowest absorbing sweeteners.

You could also occasionally consume my low-carbohydrate cheesecake. The recipe can be found at the end of this chapter.

Why don't you consider calories within this program?

Calories, which are the units of energy in foods, are rather insignificant, in my opinion, compared to the hormone influence of foods and activities. Let's take fat. Fat has high calories compared to other foods but fat does *not* stimulate fat-storing hormones. However, carbohydrates like breads or pasta can trigger fat-storing hormones. Cutting calories *can* cause long-term weight gain by stimulating the stress hormone cortisol, which releases sugar in the blood and triggers insulin to change this sugar into fat. That is why some people who go on low-calorie diets gain weight down the road.

You don't seem to put emphasis on the dangers of fats. Why?

Hydrogenated fats are bad, no doubt. But both fat-storing and fat-burning hormones treat fats as neutral, despite their having the most calories.

Is there a way to speed up getting rid of cellulite-type fat on my thighs?

This is usually an Ovary body shape. It can be one of two problems: (1) excessive estrogen or (2) fluid retention within the lymphatic system in the outer thighs. If your eyes are puffy and feel swollen, suspect lymphatic fluid retention. If you press around your bellybutton, you can usually feel some soreness due to congested lymph nodes.

The water retention situation can be solved by going on the Liver Enhancement Plan. The high potassium in these foods will balance the sodium. The key is to avoid artificial sweeteners and food chemicals and go as natural as possible. Many of these people are consuming some type of artificial sweetener within sodas or other drinks.

Fibroids and ovarian cysts can produce excess estrogen; so can HRT and birth-control pills. Growth hormones in animal meats can also contain estrogen. Make sure everything is organic and without hormones.

Another tip for this problem is to increase circulation by exercising the lower part of the body as opposed to the top part. Increasing protein in the diet can also decrease water retention. But add the protein after you have done the Liver Enhancement Plan.

I'm gaining weight on this diet. What does that mean?

It means you are building more muscle. Muscle weighs more than fat. This means your cortisol hormones have been destroying your muscle proteins. A necessary process of healing requires more protein building.

I hit a plateau and am not losing any more weight. What should I do?

After doing the Liver Enhancement Plan, some people stop losing weight when they transition to the body type diets. If this occurs, go back on the Liver Enhancement Plan for a longer time. I've had people do it for several months; this was what their livers needed.

The worse your metabolism is, the stricter your food intake needs to be. You can't afford to eat everything in moderation or even a few sweets here and there.

What might have happened as well is that you initially lost water weight, then plateaued once you started to burn fat, since fat burning is slower (one to two pounds per week). Also, look at whether your energy has increased, as this is an indicator of improvement. If it has increased, then continue; eventually the body will reach a greater level of health and the weight will come off. If your energy has not changed, then look through your diet to find what you are eating that might be preventing this. It is usually something simple like wine at night or a little bit of something sweet. One thing you have to realize is that if your diet has been bad for years, it might take some time to get your health back. I had one patient tell me, "I'm not losing and I've been eating well." I looked at her file; it was the third day of the program! You can't expect the result of 50 years of poor eating to turn around in a few days of healthy eating. Sometimes it might take eating well for several months before you achieve your ideal weight.

You could add more exercise to speed things up.

I have also created a service that might help you. It's a remote visit via the Internet. At the website you can use a Web-based program that is a companion to this book. The benefit is that you will have a trained person giving you personal supervision and analyzing your diet very closely. You'll get reports and graphs of the hormone responses to food and exercise that show if you are in fat burning or not. This program is an excellent way to give you the exact things to eat and do, based on your type, with the benefit of a personal coach. Go to http://www.fbtcoach.com/ and watch the tutorial.

My willpower is low and I'm having a hard time sticking to the program. How can I improve this?

Use the Web-based program mentioned above, which allows you to get one-on-one support. It sometimes helps to have a trained person observe everything you do and gently nudge you (or kick your butt) in the right direction.

Any tips on how I handle stress on this program?

The more stress, the more you need to add in aerobic exercise (low pulse rate, endurance), not anaerobic (high pulse rate or resistance-type). You also need to add more fat and consume zero sugars. Butter or coconut butter is an excellent food to include in the diet when you are stressed so that you can feed your adrenal hormones.

I don't have time to exercise.
Can I still lose weight on this program?

Yes, but the six fat-burning hormones have triggers; and the more you can trigger these hormones, the more weight you will lose. If you don't exercise, then you have to keep the diet really perfect. If the diet is not great, then you need to exercise more. If you're not sleeping well, then your diet and exercise need to be even better to compensate for this.

What's the best way to speed up my metabolism with exercise?

Once you graduate from the aerobic light-resistance-type exercise, you can really pick up the pace on anaerobic exercise. The key is to know that *intensity* is the most important trigger. The more intense the exercise, the more the hormone release. Do short, quick intense exercises with lots of rest in between.

I can't sleep at night. Any recommendations?

Eat four stalks of celery before bed. Celery contains active compounds called pthalides, which relax the muscles of the arteries that regulate blood pressure. Pthalides also reduce adrenal (stress) hormones, which cause high blood pressure. When researchers injected a compound derived from celery into test animals, the animals' blood pressure dropped 12–14 percent. In humans, an equivalent dose would be supplied by about four stalks of celery.*

---

* Source: George Mateljan Foundation, *The World's Healthiest Foods*: Celery.

You could also try Kombucha tea, which is a friendly bacteria and yeast product, obtainable at a health food store in the refrigerated section. It balances your pH and greatly helps sleeping. However, certain people start craving more sweet foods when they drink it, while others don't; so you'll have to judge for yourself.

Do I burn more fat when I sleep?

Fat is released via hormones, especially growth hormone. Growth hormone is active during the night while you sleep, but to get the most benefit from its fat-burning effects you should go to bed before 11:00 p.m.

Why do pain and lack of sleep keep me from weight loss?

Pain and lack of sleep trigger cortisol, which keeps you out of fat burning. If stress is keeping you from sleeping, I would recommend finding a local practitioner that I trained, in your area, to help with your pain or sleep restlessness. Go to http://www.drbergacupressure.com/.

How much water should I drink per day?

Don't ever force yourself to drink water. Drink when you are thirsty.

Is it true that consuming beef will cause cancer?

From the research I have done, a prime cause of cancer is low oxygen in the cells, which leads to alteration in the DNA and then cancer. Certain fats, called omega fatty acids, make up our cellular membranes, especially the parts that control cell respiration (breathing of oxygen). If you starve the cells of the raw materials they need in order to breathe, it seems obvious that your risk for cancer can increase. Commercial beef (grain-fed) has very low levels of omega 3 fatty acids, which are protective to your cell walls. However, when you consume grass-fed beef, omega 3 fats are much higher and hence cancer protective.

Is there a difference between farm-raised fish and wild-caught fish?

Big time! Each category has both omega 3 and omega 6 fats, which need to be in a certain ratio, but wild-caught fish have far more omega 3 fatty acids, in addition to being free of the hormones fed to farm-raised fish. So, if possible, consume wild-caught fish.

What are the benefits of broccoli sprouts?

Researchers estimate that broccoli sprouts contain *10 to 100 times the power of mature broccoli* to boost enzymes that detoxify potential carcinogens! So a healthy serving of broccoli sprouts in your salad or sandwich can offer even more protection against cancer than larger amounts of full-grown broccoli.

Broccoli sprouts are more nutritious than alfalfa sprouts. However, all sprouts contain much higher levels of nutrition than seeds and grown plants. For example, vitamin C is close to zero in seeds, whereas sprouting releases a huge amount of vitamin C.

Can I overdo eating nuts?

Yes. This is one of the most common problems, as many people stuff their bodies with nuts all day long and then feel bloated, especially when they're falling asleep. Roasted nuts and cashews usually cause the biggest problem; it's difficult to overdo walnuts or almonds. And people generally do better on raw nuts than on roasted nuts and peanut butter.

Heaviness in the abdomen, bloating or gas as a result of eating nuts is caused by the enzyme inhibitors they inherently contain. The way to handle this is to soak the nuts overnight in water to activate these enzymes and start the process of germination. (Details on how to do this are given in chapter 10, on pages 155–56.) Germinating nuts before you eat them will not only take the stress off your digestive system, it will also provide you with maximum nutrition.

Can I use spices?

Yes, but make sure they don't contain MSG. It comes in other forms: modified food starch, hydrolyzed protein, hydrolyzed vegetable protein, sodium caseinate, calcium caseinate, carrageenan, glutamic acid, yeast extract, autolyzed yeast and natural flavorings.

Avoid table salt and use sea salt.

I thought salt was bad for me; why do you recommend it for Adrenal body types?

With adrenal weakness you lose salt, so you need to replace it. Again, use sea salt, not table salt.

What do I do if I'm craving salty foods?

Add some sea salt to your diet every day until the cravings go away. This is usually indicative of adrenal weakness. Sometimes these same cases also crave licorice.

What do I do if I'm craving sweets?

Increase your fats and proteins, especially in the morning. This would be eggs (particularly the yolks), walnuts and almonds. I also recommend you eat before you get hungry, by adding snacks between meals. Craving sweets means you are burning sugar, not fat. The diet is designed to get you into fat burning so this doesn't happen.

I have developed a craving support product called CraveStopper. A couple of sprays on the tongue will eliminate nearly all taste for sweets. You will taste everything else but sweet. One application will last a few hours, and it comes in handy if you are in a pinch. It is an herbal product and has no side effects. Check it out at http://www.bergdiets.com/.

What do I do if I crave chocolate?

This is usually an adrenal or ovary weakness; serotonin deficiencies will cause people to want chocolate. Using the CraveStopper product will definitely help with this as well. When you spray it in your mouth, chocolate will taste like wax, causing you to get no pleasure from the chocolate.

Instead of eating chocolate, I would feed the adrenals by going on the Adrenal diet. If you are an addict and need to wean yourself off gradually, start with bittersweet chocolate. Another chocolate that is sweetened with Rapadura whole cane sugar is a bit better, due to the sweetener being whole sugar cane. Rapunzel makes a chocolate using this whole cane sugar, which can be purchased in health food stores and on the Internet. The advantage is that even though it's sugar, it contains all the minerals and vitamins within sugar cane and will not deplete your body.

What can I have as a sugar substitute?

The goal is to avoid all sugars, but now and then you have a birthday or other occasion where you are forced to eat some. If this occurs, the following are the best choices, listed in descending order:
- Stevia
- Agave nectar (cactus sugar)
- Raw or Tupelo honey
- Rapadura whole cane sugar
- Molasses

What about the sugar in salad dressing, gum, ketchup, etc.?

You need to start reading labels and look at the sugar amounts. It's these hidden sugars that add up to no weight loss. I get all my condiments at the health food store. Even many brands of pickles have sugar added — so read labels.

What about popcorn?

Popcorn is starch but it has fiber. You can have some occasionally; however, make sure you add real butter to slow the insulin response. If you find you are not losing weight, then cut it out.

What about puffed cereals or puffed rice cakes?

A few years ago I did an experiment on mice, using four different types of food. Each of the four groups of mice was fed either mouse food, whole-wheat bread, white bread or puffed cereal. Take a wild guess which group died first?

The puffed-cereal group died first, and then the whole-wheat group died next. Paul A. Stitt, author of *Beating the Food Giants*, mentioned that a chemical is released when the cereal is puffed, making it toxic to mice.

Avoid anything puffed.

Can't I eat whole-wheat bread?

Commercial whole-wheat bread has more chemicals and bug sprays (insecticides) than white bread because it has more nutrition for the bugs to live on. It's too much starch and it will slow your progress.

Will I ever be able to eat bread?

Once you achieve your ideal weight and size, you can add occasional bread into your diet. The kind of bread will be Ezekiel or spelt bread, as it is the least damaging to your system. Some other diet programs have several phases that gradually add the processed and refined foods back into the diet. The goal with our program is to get your body used to eating healthful foods, and then maintain that healthy eating.

Another problem with commercial bread is that not only is it too much of a starch but it is also badly processed. The flour most breads are made from loses its vitamins very soon after the grain is ground. Then synthetic vitamins are sprayed onto it. When you eat it, a depletion of these vitamins can occur. Once you achieve your ideal weight you could, in your spare time, grind some wheat fresh and make your own bread— a limited amount.

What about milk or dairy products?

Small amounts are all right to eat if the milk is organic. Cheese, cottage cheese, yogurt and kefir are okay on the Adrenal & Ovary diet. However, on the Liver & Thyroid diet, you should have smaller quantities and use low-fat or no-fat plain yogurt or cottage cheese.

Can a person consume milk, butter and cream on the program if it's all raw and unpasteurized?

Yes. If you do not have a Liver body type or gallbladder problems, a small quantity would be fine.

What about consuming soy products?

Most soy in America is genetically modified. It's in almost every product. Soy is badly processed and can increase estrogen. Occasional miso soup is okay. I heard of a man who ate so much soy he started lactating (releasing breast milk).

What about GMO foods?

Genetically modified foods are becoming a problem in the U.S. I would recommend getting a video called *The Future of Food*, which can be purchased at a video store or by going to http://www.thefutureoffood.com/.

There are four main foods that are being modified presently: corn, wheat, canola and soy. It makes you wonder if this is why so many people have allergies to these foods. Manufacturers are not currently regulated or required to mention if the food is GMO or not, which is scary. The only reason they don't want you to know is because you would not buy it.

I've heard that spinach, kale and other leafy greens produce oxalates, which make kidney stones.

This can occur if the leafy green vegetables—especially spinach—are cooked or processed. When these vegetables are eaten *raw*, the oxalic acid they contain may be beneficial in the cleansing and healing of the intestinal tract; but when they are cooked or processed, heat changes the organic (plant-based) acid into an inorganic acid that is no longer plant-based, which binds readily with calcium and other minerals to form oxalates (salts of oxalic acid). Because oxalates are not nutrients, the blood will transport them directly to the kidneys to excrete as urine. If the urine contains large amounts of calcium oxalate, this can solidify into crystals, which, in turn, contribute to the formation of kidney stones.

However, consuming apples, cranberry juice (unsweetened), apple cider vinegar, grapefruits, oranges, lemon juice and asparagus will act to counter the production of these stones. The benefits of cruciferous and other leafy green vegetables far outweigh the possibility of developing stones; and if the diet is balanced, as we recommend, and the majority of these vegetables are eaten raw, your risks are greatly lowered. But if you have stones, definitely start including the above foods and juices in your diet.

What are the benefits of cranberry juice?

Cranberries have high levels of potassium and are low in sodium, and their juice helps to support normal kidney, bladder and urinary tract functions. There is also a specific type of tannin (plant chemical) found only in cranberries and blueberries that prevents bacteria from sticking to the walls of the bladder and causing infection.

Another valuable substance found in cranberry juice is quinic acid. Because this compound does not break down in the body, it remains unchanged when excreted in the urine and its presence turns the urine acidic enough to prevent calcium from combining with oxalic or phosphoric acid to form kidney stones. In a study of persons with recurrent kidney stones, cranberry juice was found to reduce ionized calcium in their urine by more than 50 percent—very beneficial, when you consider that 75–85 percent of most kidney stones are made up of calcium salts.*

Can I continue the cranberry drink once the Liver Enhancement Plan is done?

Yes, if your body craves it. But if you do not like the cranberry drink or have to force yourself to get it down—discontinue it.

Can I continue the greens product after the Liver Enhancement?

Once you are done with the Liver Enhancement or are transitioning to a modified Liver Enhancement, you can start using the Organic Cruciferous Sprouts Food as a maintenance product. However, if you have a potbelly (Liver body type), you should stay on the Organic Cruciferous Food at 15 tablets per day until you achieve your ideal weight, as Liver types need higher doses of this supplement. Many people take the Sprouts product as a multivitamin-mineral supplement—3 to 6 per day—and those who don't eat cruciferous foods use it as a substitute for these vegetables in their diet.

What about a fruit or vegetable juice cleanse?

No way—all that concentrated juice is far too much sugar. I used to juice every day and my health started going downhill. When you eat fruits or vegetables, eat the whole thing. I will say, though, out of all the juices, carrot is the least damaging; but drinking carrot juice in such a concentrated form still gives you too much sugar.

However, there are some exceptions to juicing. For people who are very sick or have lots of fluid retention, as seen in their ankles, it is recommended that they juice fresh vegetables 1 to 2 times per day. These would include a combination of celery, carrot, beet, radish, red potato

---

* Source: George Mateljan Foundation, *The World's Healthiest Foods*: Cranberries.

and some kale. Do not store this juice in the refrigerator; it has to be consumed right away to get the full benefit of the enzymes.

What can I do for caffeine withdrawal?

Realize it will only last one to two days — three days at the most. This can happen with some people when they start the Liver Enhancement Plan, particularly if they come off coffee cold turkey. Just schedule this change when you are home over a weekend so you don't get too irritable with those around you. And if you do get grouchy at someone, don't mention my name.

What about decaffeinated coffee?

It is okay in small amounts if it's water processed and organic. Commercial decaf is filled with chemicals.

What about occasional alcoholic beverages?

Alcohol definitely sets the liver back by several days. The least damaging alcoholic beverage is low-carb light beer. The next is a white wine. Some people have the idea that drinking wine will help give them antioxidants. Yes, it may, but the damage to their livers is a bigger concern. You might also say, "People in Europe consume wine. Why can't I?" In most cases, Europeans have not been damaged by growth hormones. Their bodies are stronger and can handle small amounts of wine. If your hormone system is weak, you don't have this option yet.

How do I keep the weight off, now that I've lost it?

The goal of this program is to stabilize your organs so you can keep the weight off. The problem is not your weight; it's your hormones. This is a lifestyle change, and as you get healthier, going back to junk food won't feel right because your taste buds won't be able to tolerate much sugar.

What is the biggest reason why people gain the weight right back?

They lose weight and don't continue a good eating program long enough to achieve full stabilization of a healthy body.

Low-Carbohydrate Cheesecake

For special occasions, I've given you this recipe. With Liver body types, too many heavy fats will cause bloating—so go light.

LOW-CARBOHYDRATE CHEESECAKE RECIPE

Two 8 oz containers of cream cheese

¼ cup Tupelo honey or agave nectar

⅓ cup butter (unsalted) or ⅓ cup melted coconut butter (oil)

2 heaping tbsp peanut butter (almond butter also works well)

1 tsp vanilla extract

1⅓ cups ground nut-meal
(hazelnut, almond or pecan—I like pecan the best)

2 whole eggs

Pie dish, either glass or enamel

Overview

You will be making a nut crust with cream cheese filler, sweetened with Tupelo honey or agave nectar.

Set out two 8 oz containers of cream cheese (Philadelphia is fine) and ⅓ cup of unsalted butter or coconut butter until soft.

Making the Crust

The crust can be made from any type of nuts. You could either purchase a nut-meal (from Trader Joe's) or crush the nuts yourself.

I recommend using pecans, or Bob's Red Mill almond or hazelnut meal. Others (walnuts, cashews) can be used as well.

To crush them yourself, use a rolling pin and a cutting board. Crush into a meal (small-particle) texture.

Into a bowl, add

> 1⅓ cups of ground nut-meal
>
> ⅓ cup of soft butter or melted coconut butter
>
> 2 heaping tbsp of peanut butter or almond butter

Mix together thoroughly.

Place mixture into the pie dish. You do not have to grease the dish, due to the oils.

You need to form the crust with your fingers.

Filler

In a second bowl, add

> Two 8 oz containers of cream cheese
>
> ¼ cup of Tupelo honey or agave nectar
>
> 1 tsp of vanilla extract
>
> 2 whole eggs

Mix together either in a blender or by hand with a fork until creamy.

An additional step, which is quite good, is to sprinkle some shredded raw organic coconut over the crust, then pour the mixture onto the crust.

Preheat oven to 350 degrees and bake for 30 to 40 minutes.

A small crack should appear in the top of the cheesecake, and the top should also begin to turn a slight yellow or light brown. To assess if cooked, you could stick a fork into the center; if no residue clings to the fork, it's done.

Let set for 10 minutes to cool.

Eat away!

Acknowledgments

I would like to thank Rosemary Delderfield and Mary McCue for their excellent work in editing, copyediting and proofreading this book. They have contributed to the clarity of my message and were always one step ahead of me in completing this project. I would also like to acknowledge Allen Harris, the artist, for a fantastic job of illustrating these concepts, and Kathleen Frascella for her contribution in the testing and compiling of recipes for the book.

Glossary

acesulfame K. Sold commercially as Sunett or Sweet One, it was approved as a sugar substitute by the FDA in 1988. Acetoacetamide, a breakdown product, has been shown to affect the thyroid of rats, rabbits and dogs. This chemical may increase cancer risk in humans.

Acupressure Stress Elimination Technique (ASET). This technique is used to reduce body stress. It is an advanced form of acupressure and uses no muscle testing. Lowering body stress allows a person to have improved sleep, less muscle tightness and less body tension. Dr. Berg has observed that a large number of people have bodies stuck in stress mode, which prevents restful sleep, rejuvenation and recovery from life's hectic activities. Acupressure Stress Elimination Technique allows the muscles of the body to achieve a stable relaxed state. It is not intended to diagnose or treat any disease or medical condition.

Addison's disease. Also called adrenal insufficiency or hypocortisolism, this disease occurs when the adrenal glands do not produce enough of the hormone cortisol and, in some cases, the hormone aldosterone. It is characterized by weight loss, muscle weakness, fatigue, poor immune system, low blood pressure, and sometimes the darkening of both exposed and nonexposed skin.

adipose tissue. Fat tissue whose primary function is that of a fuel reserve or fuel storage and whose secondary function is to insulate and cushion. The brain, glands, hormones, nerves and cell walls are made of adipose tissue.

adrenal(s). The two adrenal glands sit on top of the kidneys. Their external outer portion is called the cortex, and the inner portion is called the medulla. Each area produces its own set of hormones.

adrenaline. Hormone produced by the inner part of the adrenal glands (adrenal medulla). Adrenaline has a wide range of functions. It constricts the blood vessels in some parts of the body and dilates them in others. It is involved in stress responses, maintains blood flow to all parts of the body, relaxes the smaller branches of the bronchial tubes, improving oxygen exchange, and causes shivering to generate body heat. In addition, it releases stored sugar in the body to maintain consistent energy. Also called epinephrine.

aerobic exercise. A slow-paced type of exercise (below 130 heartbeats per minute) designed to promote the supply and use of oxygen by the body. Aerobic exercise is considered endurance-type rather than intense exercise. In the first 20 to 30 minutes, stored sugar is used as fuel; after 30 minutes, fat can be tapped into. *Aerobic* in this context means "with oxygen." It derives from the Greek *aer*, "air," and *bios*, "life," + *-ic*, meaning "produced by" or "caused by."

agave nectar. Natural low-calorie sweetener that comes from the cactus plant. It is a stronger sweetener than sugar yet is absorbed into the bloodstream even more slowly than honey.

amino acids. The building blocks of protein. Twenty amino acids are needed to build the various proteins used in the growth, repair and maintenance of body tissues. Eleven of these, the *nonessential amino acids*, can be manufactured by the body, whereas the other nine—known as *essential amino acids*—must come from food. Amino acids form the raw material for a number of hormones. Some amino acids trigger fat-burning hormones (e.g., growth hormone).

anaerobic exercise. An intense resistance-type exercise that involves a higher pulse rate (greater than 145 heartbeats per minute). During the workout, energy is produced without utilizing oxygen and the only source of fuel is sugar in the blood or stored sugar in the muscles and liver. Fat is not burned while exercising; however, fat-burning hormones are stimulated 14 to 48 hours later. *Anaerobic* means "without oxygen"—from the Greek *an-*, "without," *aer*, "air," and *bios*, "life," + *-ic*, meaning "produced by" or "caused by."

androgens. Hormones produced by several glands (adrenals, testicles and ovaries), which are responsible for the male characteristics. *Andro-* means "man" + *-gen*, "something that produces."

anticarcinogenic. Fights, prevents or blocks cancer. Cruciferous vegetables have anticarcinogenic properties.

antiestrogenic. Inhibits or blocks estrogen. Certain cruciferous vegetables have this effect because they help the liver detoxify estrogen.

anti-inflammatory. "Against inflammation"—suppressing or reducing inflammation. The adrenal glands produce hormones that have anti-inflammatory effects.

ascites. A condition involving accumulation of fluid in the abdominal sac (tissue surrounding abdominal organs). Ascites can be caused by a failing liver, kidney or pancreas.

ascorbic acid. Part of the vitamin C complex known as the antioxidant portion.

aspartame. Artificial sweetener marketed under a number of trademark names, such as NutraSweet and Equal; it is an ingredient in approximately 6,000 consumer foods and beverages sold worldwide. Several thousand reports have been submitted to the FDA by both patients and doctors, complaining of 92 different adverse health effects attributed to aspartame.*

---

* Department of Health and Human Services. "Adverse Reactions Associated with Aspartame Consumption." HFS-728, 1993 (April 1).

atrophy. Breakdown and shrinkage of an organ, gland or muscle, which can occur as a result of excessive hormone secretion, such as cortisol.

autoimmunity. A condition in which the body produces antibodies that attack its own cells and tissues. Normally, adrenal hormones are supposed to suppress immune cells, but when this function is broken, the immune system can go out of control. Autoimmune diseases result from a hyperactive immune system attacking normal tissues as if they were foreign organisms.

autolyze. To undergo, or cause to undergo, autolysis—the destruction of cells or tissues by an organism's own enzymes, as after a disease or death. Also called *self-digestion*. Autolysis is used as a method of producing yeast extract.

biopsy. The removal of bits of tissue from a living body for examination.

calorie. Derived from the Latin word *calor*, meaning "heat," calorie refers to the amount of energy in a food. Different foods of the same quantity contain higher or lower amounts of energy (calories).

Candida. A yeast-like fungus that is normally in balance with other friendly microbes. However, an overgrowth of Candida can occur after antibiotic use.

capillary. Any of the tiny blood vessels that connect the smallest arteries with the smallest veins.

carbohydrate. Any of a group of substances made of carbon, hydrogen and oxygen, including the sugars, fibers and starches, used by the body as an energy source. There are several types of carbohydrates: grains, vegetables, fruits and sugars. Unrefined carbohydrates provide vitamins and minerals as well as fiber, while refined grains, in the form of breads, pasta, cereals, crackers, donuts and the like, have little nutrient value.

carcinogen. A substance that causes or is capable of causing cancer. Examples are pesticides, insecticides, herbicides, fungicides, plastics, solvents and heavy metals.

carrageenan. A thickening compound extracted from seaweed and red algae, used in some dairy products to stabilize the color and flavor. It often contains MSG and has been linked to digestive upset.

cartilage: Tough elastic tissue assisting in the support of joints.

caseinate. A chemical made from milk protein (casein) and used to stabilize certain foods.

cholesterol. A substance that occurs in egg yolks, meats and dairy products. It is also made by the liver and many other body cells and is an important raw material in the production of hormones. Cholesterol supplies the material to make nerves, brain tissue and endocrine tissue. It also allows nerve transmission, healing and immune system functions. Seventy-five percent of the cholesterol in the body is made by the liver and cells; only 25 percent comes from outside dietary sources. Excessively low cholesterol can weaken the immune system. LDL (bad cholesterol) is a term used to describe the cholesterol going into the liver. HDL (good cholesterol) is a term describing cholesterol coming out of the liver.

circadian rhythm. A rhythmic cycle in the body that occurs roughly every 24 hours. Linked to the light-dark cycle, circadian rhythms are important in determining the sleeping and feeding patterns of all animals, including human beings. Patterns of brain-wave activity, hormone production, cell regeneration and other biological activities are also connected to this daily cycle. The term *circadian* comes from the Latin *circa*, "about," and *dies*, "day," meaning literally "about a day."

cirrhosis. Chronic condition of the liver in which normal tissue is replaced by fibrous scar tissue and normal function is inhibited.

collagen. The main structural protein found in skin, ligaments, tendons, bone, cartilage and other connective tissue. It is the most abundant protein in mammals, making up about 25 percent of the total protein content. Collagen consists of groups of strong white inelastic fibers, enabling these body structures to withstand forces that stretch them. Since it is responsible for skin strength and elasticity, its deterioration leads to wrinkles that accompany aging. Derived from French *collagène*, from Greek *kola*, "glue," + *-gen*, "something that produces," the word *collagen* means "glue producer" and refers to the early process of boiling the skin and sinews of horses and other animals to obtain glue.

cortisol. Important hormone produced by the adrenal glands to counter stress responses. It is anti-inflammatory and releases glucose from the liver and muscles into the blood to help the body respond to stress. It also suppresses immune cells (white blood cells) and is involved in sleep cycles. Cortisol is an indirect fat-making hormone; when it releases excess glucose into the blood, this causes abnormally high insulin levels to convert the sugar into fat around the abdominal organs.

cruciferous. A group of vegetables belonging to the cabbage family, which includes cabbage, bok choy, collards, broccoli, Brussels sprouts, kohlrabi, kale, mustard greens, turnip greens and cauliflower. These leafy green vegetables contain more phytochemicals (plant chemicals) than any other food, which may strengthen the immune system and thereby help build resistance against viruses and diseases. The term is derived from the Latin word *crux*, meaning "cross," because the four petals of these plants' tiny flowers resemble a cross.

cyst. A sac-like structure in plants and animals. In certain abnormal conditions, this sac becomes filled with fluid or disease matter.

delta-wave sleep. Slow-wave or deep sleep, which occurs mostly in the first third of the night. A delta wave is a large, slow electrical brain wave, marking the deepest level of sleep.

detoxification. The removal of poisons or toxins from the body.

diastolic. Refers to when the heart is in a period of relaxation and dilation (expansion). In a blood pressure reading the diastolic pressure is the second number recorded. For example, if the reading is 120/80, the bottom number is the diastolic measurement. By "80" is meant 80 mm of mercury. This number measures the pressure against the blood vessel walls when the heart is between beats and resting. Derived from the Greek *diastol*, "expansion," "dilation," from *dia*, "apart" + *stellein*, "to put." See also **systolic**.

diet. 1. The usual food and drink consumed by a person or animal. 2. A regulated course of food and drink to promote health or for weight control. The word *diet* comes from the Old French *diète*, from Latin *diaeta*, which means "way of living."

diethylstilbestrol (DES). A type of synthetic estrogen used in the 1940s through to the 1960s as a growth hormone to fatten meat-producing animals. It was also given to pregnant women to prevent miscarriages but is now banned because it was found to cause both cancer and birth abnormalities.

diuretic. A substance (medication or food) that rids the body of excess fluid by increasing the flow of urine.

edema. Swelling of tissues in the body caused by an abnormal accumulation of fluid.

electrolyte(s). A large category of substances—which include sodium, potassium, calcium, magnesium, chloride and bicarbonate—whose water solution will carry an electric current. Cells use electrolytes to transmit electrical impulses (nerve impulses, muscle contractions) across themselves and to other cells. These chemicals are essential in many bodily processes, such as fluid balance, nerve conduction, muscle function (including heartbeat), blood clotting and pH balance.

endocrine disruptor. An environmental poison that mimics, blocks or otherwise disrupts the normal function of hormones. It is an exogenous (coming from outside the body) substance that changes endocrine function and can cause adverse developmental and reproductive effects in living organisms and their offspring, as well as being a potential carcinogen in the environment. Examples include pesticides, insecticides, herbicides, fungicides, plastics, solvents and heavy metals.

endocrine system. The entire collection of glands that produce and release hormones; together these glands and hormones influence almost every cell, organ and function of the body. The system as a whole communicates through the blood vessels and lymphatic system. Hormones are sent from one gland to another, or to a remote tissue, creating some effect. The characteristic feature of the endocrine glands is that they are ductless (without ducts). Because the liver does have a duct (bile duct connection to the small intestine), it is not considered a true endocrine gland even though it produces a hormone. This system is the body's main communication system. The term *endocrine* is derived from the Greek words *endon*, "within," and *krinein*, "to separate."

enzyme. A protein substance produced by all living plants and animals that both causes and greatly increases the speed of chemical reactions. Found in every organ of the body, enzymes cause specific chemical changes without being used up or chemically altered themselves. Enzymes are known to catalyze about 4,000 biochemical reactions. For instance, the liver produces enzymes to break down toxic chemicals into harmless substances; other enzymes change starches, proteins and sugars into material the body can digest; blood clotting is another example. Without enzymes, chemical reactions would be very slow.

epinephrine. See **adrenaline**.

estrogen: A general name for the female sex hormone produced by the ovaries. There are three main naturally occurring estrogens in women: estradiol, estriol and estrone. These are responsible for the female characteristics, menstrual cycle, and changes of the uterus and breasts; they also provide the fat layer around the female body. Derived from the Greek *oistros*, "mad desire," and *genēs*, "born."

fat (dietary). Provides essential fatty acids for growth and development of body tissue, as well as fat-soluble vitamins. Essential fatty acids are fats that must come from the diet—flax or fish oil, nuts, olives, avocados, vegetables (or their oils) and seeds. The body can also make some of the fats it needs from carbohydrates.

fibromyalgia. An inflammatory condition that affects many muscles, joints and connective tissues in the body.

genetically modified organisms (GMOs). Organisms that have had their genes manipulated (1) to introduce new, or alter existing, characteristics or (2) to produce a new protein or enzyme. Genetic modification is used to increase the yield or quality of various crops.

gland. An organ or structure whose secretions include hormones, mucus and sweat. Derived from the Latin *glans*, meaning "acorn."

glucagon. The opposing hormone to insulin, glucagon raises blood sugar and is a fat-burning hormone. It helps regulate blood sugar between meals and is stimulated by proteins and intense exercise.

glucose. The simplest form of sugar and carbohydrate. The body uses hormones to change body proteins into sugar and stores glucose in the liver and muscles as glycogen.

glutamic acid. A nonessential amino acid that occurs widely in plant and animal tissue and is used by the body to build proteins. It is supplied by most food sources of protein. Glutamate, a salt of glutamic acid, has a stimulating effect on the central nervous system. Monosodium glutamate (MSG) is a form of glutamic acid used as a flavor enhancer.

gluten. The protein part of wheat.

GMO. See **genetically modified organisms**.

growth hormone (GH). A fat-burning, lean-muscle-building hormone that contributes to growth. GH rebuilds body tissue, including joints, bones and muscles; it also builds up cartilage and collagen. It is an antiaging hormone. Growth hormone works through the liver; it regulates fuel between meals and is active during the sleep cycle.

hormone. A chemical message that originates in an organ or gland and is sent through the blood or lymph to another part of the body, triggering an increase or decrease in function. Hormones are made from cholesterol, amino acids, fatty acids and protein. Functions include burning fat, storing fat, the regulation of sleep cycles, blood pressure, cholesterol levels, hair growth, and changes in the menstrual cycle. Hormones also control the reproductive cycle of virtually all multicellular organisms. There are several hundred hormones and each one has a different action and effect. Environmental chemicals and toxins can also mimic, block, alter and confuse hormones. Derived from the Greek *hormon*, from *horman*, "to set in motion."

hormone-free animal products. Products from animals raised without added hormones.

hormone receptor. A sensor tissue in the body that receives hormonal messages. Receptors can be on the cells' surface or within the cells.

hormone replacement therapy (HRT). A synthetic blend of the hormone estrogen and progestin (a synthetic form of progesterone), used to replace hormones the female body no longer produces after menopause. Studies show that side effects include stroke, cancer, and possibly heart disease. There are conflicting data on whether HRT is beneficial or harmful to the heart.

hydrogenate. To combine a fluid oil with hydrogen in order to produce a solid fat.

hydrolyze. To subject to hydrolysis—a chemical process in which a substance reacts to water so as to be changed from one thing into another, such as a starch to glucose or a fat into fatty acids or a protein into its component amino acids. In protein powders, hydrolyzing is a form of predigesting the protein to make it absorb more easily when eaten. Hydrolyzed proteins are also proteins from certain foods that have been treated with an acid or enzyme and are then used in the same manner as MSG in products such as canned vegetables, soups and processed meats.

hypothalamus. A master gland in the brain that controls homeostasis (the body's ability to adapt to environmental changes and maintain normal stability of its internal functions—temperature, blood sugar, blood pressure, etc.).

hypothesis. A tentative explanation for an observation, phenomenon or scientific problem that needs to be tested by further investigation.

immune system. The body's defense mechanism against disease, infection and foreign substances. It is made up of highly specialized cells, tissues and organs, with a circulatory system separate from blood vessels, all of which work together to protect the body. The special circulatory system carries lymph, a transparent fluid containing white blood cells whose function is to seek out and destroy the organisms or substances that cause disease. See also **lymphatic system.**

insulin: Hormone produced by the pancreas that lowers blood sugar after meals to maintain normal blood sugars and prevent high blood sugar levels. Insulin will cause the cells to absorb sugar as fuel and will convert the rest to fat and cholesterol.

insulin-like growth factor (IGF). Hormone made by the liver that regulates blood sugars between meals. It releases stored sugar and fat, maintaining blood glucose at a normal level. Insulin and IGF work in tandem to keep blood sugars in balance.

insulin resistance: A condition where the insulin receptors on the surface of the cells won't let insulin be accepted, causing the pancreas to secrete higher amounts of insulin. When the body cells resist or do not respond even to high levels of insulin, glucose builds up in the blood creating a type 2 diabetes situation.

iodized salt. Salt that has iodine added to it. Used primarily to prevent thyroid problems.

ion. An atom or group of atoms that are normally electrically neutral and become electrically charged during a chemical reaction.

isolate. A dry powder food ingredient—such as soy protein isolate or whey protein isolate—that has been separated, or isolated, from the other components of the soybean, whey, etc., making it 90 to 95 percent protein and nearly carbohydrate and fat free.

ketosis. Ketones are a normal byproduct of fat metabolism (the breaking down of fat into energy). When ketones are in the urine, it means the body is breaking down fat. There are two types of ketosis: (1) *dietary ketosis*, which is the body's normal reaction when a person consumes primarily or only fat and protein, thus forcing the body to burn fat; (2) *ketoacidosis*, which is a dangerous condition for diabetics and is considered a disease, where the blood pH becomes overly acidic due to extremely high blood glucose, and ketones are produced by the body to provide the fuel necessary for life, since the sugar cannot be utilized because of the diabetes.

lactic acid. A waste product of sugar metabolism. The body generates lactic acid when stored sugar is burned from the muscles and liver. The body can also use lactic acid as a fuel source, burning it in a way similar to the way it burns a sugar fuel. The body will utilize sugar and lactic acid as fuel before it uses fat as fuel.

lecithin. A substance that helps break down fats and cholesterol. Lecithin is present in eggs and other foods that contain fat. It is considered anticholesterol.

lymphatic system. A major part of the immune system, it helps defend the body against viruses, bacteria and fungi that can cause illnesses. Its three main functions are maintaining fluid balance in the body, immunity, and the absorption and transport of fatty acids from the small intestine to the blood. The system is made up of a network of lymphatic vessels, which carry lymph (a clear, watery fluid containing the disease-fighting white blood cells as well as salts, glucose and other substances) throughout the body;

lymph nodes—small masses of tissue located along the lymph vessels, which house a type of white blood cell and filter out destroyed microorganisms; and lymph organs, including the bone marrow, spleen, thymus gland and tonsils. The word *lymph* comes from the French *lymphe*, from Latin *lympha*, meaning "clear water." See also **immune system**.

metabolic rate. The rate at which the body utilizes energy. This rate is controlled by hormones. The thyroid gland is a very important factor in metabolic rate.

metabolism. The sum of the physical and chemical changes that occur in the body, necessary for the maintenance of life. Examples are the breaking down of food to produce energy and the utilization of that energy to perform vital life functions; and the breakdown of fat and stored sugar, yielding fuel to power other bodily activities. Metabolism involves two processes: (1) the building up of tissue (anabolism), as occurs in bone or muscle growth, and (2) the breaking down of tissue (catabolism), as in the release of fat from the reserves or the breakdown of muscle tissue after exercise. Metabolism is influenced by hormones. The term derives from the Greek word *metabolē*, "change," + *-ism*, meaning "the condition of."

mitochondria. Very small, usually rod-like structures found in the cells, which act as energy factories to regulate metabolism. Fat and sugar are turned into energy by the mitochondria, and the thyroid gland controls their number and size.

myxedema. A skin and tissue disorder caused by an extreme deficiency of thyroid hormone. It is characterized by dry, thickening skin and a swelling of the skin and other tissues, particularly around the eyes, lips and nose. The swelling is not a true form of fat, but rather a wastelike substance that accumulates between the cells. Fluid is trapped as well. Because of its spongelike nature, the excess fluid remains immobile, and the edema is nonpitting— that is, if pressure is applied to the skin, it does not result in a persistent indentation. Derived from the Greek *myxa*, "mucus" or "slime," and *oidēma*, "swelling."

nitrates. Refers to sodium nitrate—a chemical used to preserve and color food, especially meat and fish products; implicated in the formation of suspected carcinogens.

organic. 1. Grown with only animal or vegetable fertilizers, such as manure, bone meal or compost, and without the use of chemical fertilizers, pesticides, fungicides, herbicides or insecticides. 2. Plant-based; derived from living organisms. Plants take rocks from the soil—calcium carbonate, iron ore, copper—and change these inorganic minerals to plant-based (organic) minerals, making the bonds between the molecules weaker and thus easier for the body to break down. [Note: These definitions apply to the use of *organic* within this book. Further definitions can be found in a dictionary.]

pH. A symbol used (with a number) to indicate acidity or alkalinity. It represents the concentration of hydrogen ions in a given solution. On the pH scale, values range from 0 to 14. A pH of 7 is considered neutral. Pure water has a pH of 7. Substances with a pH value above 7 are alkaline; those with a pH below 7 are acidic. The term derives from German: *p* stands for *Potenz*, meaning "potency" or "power," and *H* is the symbol for hydrogen, the ion that determines acidity or alkalinity.

pituitary. A gland in the brain that acts as a relay between the hypothalamus and other glands (ovaries, adrenals, liver, thyroid and testes).

polycystic ovarian syndrome (PCOS). A condition where multiple small cysts form in the ovaries (*poly* means "many"), related to the ovary's failure to release an egg. PCOS can create facial hair, weight gain, insulin resistance and a disruption in the menstrual cycle.

protein. One of the three types of nutrients used by the body as energy sources, the other two being carbohydrate and fat. Its building blocks are amino acids. The body's cells are composed of 50 percent protein. Protein is needed for growth and development and is used by the body to make muscles, organs, glands, skin, bone, hair, nails, blood and the immune system; even body fluids (except bile and urine) contain protein. See also **amino acids**.

Ragland's test. A blood pressure test used to indicate the general health of the adrenal glands, which provides information on how the adrenals respond to stress. The blood pressure is first taken when a person has been lying down for a few minutes. It is then taken a second time, immediately after the person stands up. In a normal reading, the top number (systolic) is from 6 to 10 points higher when the person is standing than when he or she is lying down. A rise of 0 to 5 points indicates a borderline adrenal problem, while a drop gives a relative indication of diminished adrenal function.

saccharin. The oldest-known artificial sweetener, it is a white crystalline powder produced from coal tar, having a taste about 500 times sweeter than cane sugar but with a slightly bitter metallic aftertaste. The sodium or calcium salt of saccharin is widely used as a calorie-free sweetener in special dietary foods and beverages and to improve the taste of pharmaceuticals, toothpaste and other toiletries; it is also used as a sugar substitute in diabetic diets.

serotonin. A hormone found in the brain, blood and digestive tract, which allows nerve cells throughout the body to communicate and interact with each other. It helps smooth muscles to contract, such as the abdominal muscles that aid digestion, and also plays a part in regulating the expansion and contraction of blood vessels, assisting in the clotting of blood to close a wound. Some of the body's serotonin is produced by the adrenal glands, and its presence in the body creates a sense of well-being or comfort.

Splenda. Also known as sucralose, it is an artificial sweetener derived from chlorinated sucrose (table sugar). It is 320-1,000 times sweeter than sucrose. While there are no long-term human studies for sucralose, animal studies have shown shrunken thymus glands (up to 40 percent shrinkage), enlarged liver and kidneys, atrophy of lymph follicles in the spleen and thymus, reduced growth rate, decreased red blood cell count, aborted pregnancy, decreased placental and fetal body weights, and diarrhea.

steroids. Any of numerous natural or synthetic fat-soluble compounds, including many hormones, body components (e.g., cholesterol, bile acids, and the adrenal and sex hormones) and drugs. Steroid hormones such as cortisol or cortisone are anti-inflammatory hormones produced by the adrenal glands.

stevia. A herb or shrub of the same family as sunflowers, its extracts have up to 300 times the sweetness of sugar.

sulfite. A type of food preservative, often found in wines, dried fruits and dried potato products, and sometimes added to bottled juices, pickles and other food items.

sympathetic nervous system. Part of the nervous system that prepares the body for physical action, emergency or sudden stress. The heartbeat accelerates, blood sugar rises, perspiration occurs, digestion is slowed, blood flow to the skin is decreased, and arteries are dilated, increasing blood flow to the muscles. This process is known as the body's fight-or-flight response.

synthetic vitamins. Vitamins manufactured from chemicals (mostly coal-tar products) as compared with whole vitamin complexes found in nature that come from plant and animal sources. They are isolated parts of the vitamins that occur naturally in food, and they not only cannot perform the same functions in the body as natural whole vitamin complexes but in many cases can be harmful to the system.

systolic. The blood pressure when the heart is contracting. In a blood pressure reading, the systolic pressure is the first number recorded. For example, if the reading is 120/80, the top number of 120 is the systolic measurement. By "120" is meant 120 mm of mercury. This number measures the pressure against the blood vessel walls when the heart is pumping blood to the organs. Derived from the Greek *systolē*, from *systellein*, "to draw together." See also **diastolic**.

testosterone. A steroid hormone from the androgen group. Testosterone is secreted primarily in the testicles of males and the ovaries of females, although small amounts are secreted by the adrenal glands. It is the principal male sex hormone. In both males and females, it plays key roles in health and well-being. Examples include enhanced libido, energy, immune function, and protection against osteoporosis.

trans fats. Also known as trans fatty acids and hydrogenated or partially hydrogenated fats, these are man-made or processed fats, produced by adding hydrogen gas to a liquid fat or oil to make it thicker or more solid. This increases its shelf life, as it is less likely to spoil. Hydrogenating the oil in peanut butter, for instance, gives the product a creamy consistency and prevents the oil from rising to the top. However, trans fats are very hard on the liver, and consuming them can contribute to an increase in total cholesterol as well as a drop in the good cholesterol. They also increase the risk of heart disease. Trans fats can be found in numerous foods, including commercially prepared baked goods, some commercially fried foods, packaged snacks, cakes, cookies, crackers, peanut butter, stick margarine and vegetable shortening. Harvard School of Public Health estimates there are 30,000 American deaths each year from eating trans fats, making these fats silent killers.*

triglycerides. Blood fats.

Tupelo honey. A slow-absorbing honey that is recommended to diabetics.

virus. A portion of genetic material wrapped in protein. Viruses can reproduce only by invading and taking over other cells because they lack the cellular machinery for self-reproduction. They are parasitic, which means they live off the energy from other cells. People become susceptible to viruses when their resistance is lowered. Viruses can be sent into remission (inactivation).

---

* http://www.udoerasmus.com/articles/udo/trans_fats_labelling.htm

vitamins. A group of compounds needed in small amounts by the body to maintain health and normal functioning. Vitamins are obtained from food, and some are made by the body. They are not used by the body as fuel but rather as cofactors and regulators of cell function. (A *cofactor* is an accessory substance that must be present for a particular biological reaction to occur.) Derived from the Latin *vita*, which means "life," + *amine*, because vitamins were originally thought to contain amino acids.

vitamins K and J. Vitamin K is a fat-soluble vitamin that promotes blood clotting; vitamin J is the anti-pneumonia factor. Normally these two vitamins work synergistically with vitamin C.

References

For complete documentation on the authors and publications cited below, refer to the bibliography on pages 309–11. If you would like a copy of any of the references, write to quickquestion@bergdiets.com.

CHAPTER 2: *The 7 Principles of Fat Burning*

1. Netter, *CIBA Collection of Medical Illustrations*, Vol. 4, 101.

   Bacon and Di Bisceglie, *Liver Disease*, 24.

2. Gillette, Bullough, and Melby, "Postexercise Energy Expenditure," 347–60.

   Schuenke, Mikat, and McBride, "Post-Exercise Oxygen Consumption," 411–17.

CHAPTER 3: *Hormones and Your Body Shape*

1. Netter, *CIBA Collection of Medical Illustrations*, Vol. 4, 121.

2. U.S. EPA, "Endocrine Disruptors Research Initiative," http://www.epa.gov/endocrine/.

3. Univ. of Wisconsin, "Endocrine Disrupters," http://whyfiles.org/045env_hormone/main1.html.

4. Berkson, *Hormone Deception*, 218.

5. Klaassen, *Casarett & Doull's Toxicology*, 16.

CHAPTER 5: *The Adrenal Type*

1. Guyton, *Textbook of Medical Physiology*, 916.

2. Netter, *CIBA Collection of Medical Illustrations*, Vol. 4, 85.

3. Guyton, *Textbook of Medical Physiology*, 916.

4. Guyton, *Textbook of Medical Physiology*, 822.

   Guyton, *Textbook of Medical Physiology*, 823.

5. Guyton, *Textbook of Medical Physiology*, 914.

   Guyton, *Textbook of Medical Physiology*, 817.

6. Netter, *CIBA Collection of Medical Illustrations*, Vol. 4, 86.

7. Netter, *CIBA Collection of Medical Illustrations*, Vol. 4, 87.

8. Netter, *CIBA Collection of Medical Illustrations*, Vol. 4, 87.

9. Netter, *CIBA Collection of Medical Illustrations*, Vol. 4, 85.

10. Netter, *CIBA Collection of Medical Illustrations*, Vol. 4, 86.

11. Netter, *CIBA Collection of Medical Illustrations*, Vol. 4, 87.

12. Guyton, *Textbook of Medical Physiology*, 917.

CHAPTER 7: *The Thyroid Type*

1. Guyton, *Textbook of Medical Physiology*, 816.

2. Guyton, *Textbook of Medical Physiology*, 902–03.

3. Lee, *About Menopause*, 147.

4. Shomon, *Living Well with Hypothyroidism*, 268.

5. Guyton, *Textbook of Medical Physiology*, 907.

6. Colborn, Dumanoski, and Myers, *Our Stolen Future*, 40.

CHAPTER 8: *The Liver Type*

1. Bacon and Di Bisceglie, *Liver Disease*, 21.

2. Netter, *CIBA Collection of Medical Illustrations*, Vol. 3, 84.
   Netter, *CIBA Collection of Medical Illustrations*, Vol. 3, 97.

3. Netter, *CIBA Collection of Medical Illustrations*, Vol. 4, 71.

4. Netter, *CIBA Collection of Medical Illustrations*, Vol. 3, 70.

5. Netter, *CIBA Collection of Medical Illustrations*, Vol. 3, 71.

6. Netter, *CIBA Collection of Medical Illustrations*, Vol. 4, 156.

7. Bacon and Di Bisceglie, *Liver Disease*, 24–28.

8. Netter, *CIBA Collection of Medical Illustrations*, Vol. 3, 42.

9. Netter, *CIBA Collection of Medical Illustrations*, Vol. 4, 212.

10. Faigin, *Natural Hormonal Enhancement*, 201.

11. Faigin, *Natural Hormonal Enhancement*, 6.

12. Faigin, *Natural Hormonal Enhancement*, 8.

Chapter 9: The 10 Fat-Burning Triggers and Blockers

Trigger #1—The Absence of Sugar

1. Guyton, *Textbook of Medical Physiology*, 823.

2. Guyton, *Textbook of Medical Physiology*, 926.

   Guyton, *Textbook of Medical Physiology*, 930.

   Guyton, *Textbook of Medical Physiology*, 820.

   Guyton, *Textbook of Medical Physiology*, 819.

   Guyton, *Textbook of Medical Physiology*, 822.

3. Guyton, *Textbook of Medical Physiology*, 927.

   Guyton, *Textbook of Medical Physiology*, 824.

   Guyton, *Textbook of Medical Physiology*, 822.

   Guyton, *Textbook of Medical Physiology*, 927.

   Guyton, *Textbook of Medical Physiology*, 930.

   Guyton, *Textbook of Medical Physiology*, 927.

4. Guyton, *Textbook of Medical Physiology*, 931.

   Guyton, *Textbook of Medical Physiology*, 931.

   Guyton, *Textbook of Medical Physiology*, 823.

   Griffin and Ojeda, *Endocrine Physiology*, 396.

Guyton, *Textbook of Medical Physiology*, 823.

5. Faigin, *Natural Hormonal Enhancement*, 239.

6. Guyton, *Textbook of Medical Physiology*, 930.

Guyton, *Textbook of Medical Physiology*, 932.

7. Guyton, *Textbook of Medical Physiology*, 930.

Guyton, *Textbook of Medical Physiology*, 931.

Trigger #2—Vegetables

8. Medical College of Wisconsin, "Very High Fiber Diet," http://healthlink.mcw.edu/article/958073584.html.

Trigger #3 — Protein

9. Guyton, *Textbook of Medical Physiology*, 837.

Guyton, *Textbook of Medical Physiology*, 833.

Guyton, *Textbook of Medical Physiology*, 837.

10. Guyton, *Textbook of Medical Physiology*, 889.

Guyton, *Textbook of Medical Physiology*, 932.

Guyton, *Textbook of Medical Physiology*, 932.

11. Guyton, *Textbook of Medical Physiology*, 862.

12. Guyton, *Textbook of Medical Physiology*, 862.

Trigger #4—Fats

13. Guyton, *Textbook of Medical Physiology*, 825.

Griffin and Ojeda, *Endocrine Physiology*, 404.

14. Lewis et al., "Effect of Diet Composition," 160–70.

15. Netter, *CIBA Collection of Medical Illustrations*, Vol. 3, 52.

    Colorado State University, "Cholecystokinin,"
    http://www.vivo.colostate.edu./hbooks/pathphys/endocrine/gi/cck.html.

16. Guyton, *Textbook of Medical Physiology*, 822.

    Netter, *CIBA Collection of Medical Illustrations*, Vol. 3, 37.

    Yancy et al., "Low-Carbohydrate, Ketogenic Diet," 769–77.

    Achten and Jeukendrup, "Optimizing Fat Oxidation," 723.

**Trigger #5—Skipping Meals, Reducing Calories or
Letting Yourself Get Hungry**

17. Guyton, *Textbook of Medical Physiology*, 817.

Trigger #6 — Gland Destroyers

18. Bacon and Di Bisceglie, *Liver Disease*, 24.

    Bacon and Di Bisceglie, *Liver Disease*, 25.

19. Lane et al., "Caffeine Effects," 320–36.

Trigger #8 — Exercise

20. Faigin, *Natural Hormonal Enhancement*, 238–40.

21. Faigin, *Natural Hormonal Enhancement*, 242.

22. Nicklas, *Endurance Exercise and Adipose Tissue*, 5.

23. Guyton, *Textbook of Medical Physiology*, 889, fig. 75-5.

    Guyton, *Textbook of Medical Physiology*, 930.

    Guyton, *Textbook of Medical Physiology*, 930.

Guyton, *Textbook of Medical Physiology*, 932.

Guyton, *Textbook of Medical Physiology*, 824.

Trigger #9 — Stress

24. Guyton, *Textbook of Medical Physiology*, 918.

Netter, *CIBA Collection of Medical Illustrations*, Vol. 4, 85.

Trigger #10 — Sleep

25. Guyton, *Textbook of Medical Physiology*, 889.

26. Netter, *CIBA Collection of Medical Illustrations*, Vol. 4, 87.

27. Faigin, *Natural Hormonal Enhancement*, 201.

CHAPTER 14: *Exercising for Your Body Type*

1. Guyton, *Textbook of Medical Physiology*, 932.

2. Guyton, *Textbook of Medical Physiology,* 932.

3. Schuenke, Mikat, and McBride, "Post-Exercise Oxygen Consumption," 411–17.

Bibliography

Achten, Juul, and Asker E. Jeukendrup. "Optimizing Fat Oxidation Through Exercise and Diet." *Nutrition* 20, nos. 7/8 (2004): 716–27.

Bacon, Bruce R., and Adrian M. Di Bisceglie, eds. *Liver Disease: Diagnosis* and *Management*. Philadelphia: Churchill Livingstone, 2000.

Berkson, D. Lindsey. *Hormone Deception*. Chicago: Contemporary Books, 2000.

Brassica Protection Products LLC.
http://www.brassica.com/sci/patents.htm.
http://www.broccosprouts.com/sprouts/story.htm.

Cherniske, Stephen. *Caffeine Blues: Wake Up to the Hidden Dangers of America's #1 Drug*. New York: Warner Books, 1998.

Colborn, Theo, Dianne Dumanoski, and John Peterson Myers. *Our Stolen Future*. New York: Plume, 1997.

Colorado State University. "Pathophysiology of the Endocrine System: Gastrointestinal Hormones: Cholecystokinin." *Hypertexts for Biomedical Sciences*.
http://www.vivo.colostate.edu./hbooks/pathphys/endocrine/gi/cck.html.

Crickenberger, Roger G., and Roy E. Carawan. "Using Food Processing By-Products for Animal Feed." *Water Quality and Waste Management*, North Carolina Cooperative Extension Service, 1996.
http://www.bae.ncsu.edu/programs/extension/publicat/wqwm/cd37.html.

Faigin, Rob. *Natural Hormonal Enhancement*. Cedar Mountain, NC: Extique, 2000.

George Mateljan Foundation. *The World's Healthiest Foods.* http://www.whfoods.org/foodstoc.php.

Gillette, C. A., R. C. Bullough, and C. L. Melby. "Postexercise Energy Expenditure in Response to Acute Aerobic or Resistive Exercise." *Int J Sport Nutr* 4, no. 4 (1994): 347–60.

Griffin, James E., and Sergio R. Ojeda, eds. *Textbook of Endocrine Physiology.* 4th ed. New York: Oxford University Press, 2000.

Guyton, Arthur C. *Textbook of Medical Physiology.* 7th ed. Philadelphia: W. B. Saunders, 1986.

Kirby, Alex. "Waste 'Was Fed to UK Cattle.'" *BBC News*, October 27, 1999. http://news.bbc.co.uk/1/hi/sci/tech/486421.stm.

Klaassen, Curtis D., ed. *Casarett & Doull's Toxicology: The Basic Science of Poisons.* 6th ed. New York: McGraw-Hill, 2001.

Lane, J. D., R. A. Adcock, R. B. Williams, and C. M. Kuhn. "Caffeine Effects on Cardiovascular and Neuroendocrine Responses to Acute Psychosocial Stress and Their Relationship to Level of Habitual Caffeine Consumption." *Psychosom Med* 52, no. 3 (1990): 320–36.

Lee, John R. *What Your Doctor May Not Tell You about Menopause.* With Virginia Hopkins. New York: Warner Books, 1996.

Lewis, S. B., J. D. Wallin, J. P. Kane, and J. E. Gerich. "Effect of Diet Composition on Metabolic Adaptations to Hypocaloric Nutrition: Comparison of High Carbohydrate and High Fat Isocaloric Diets." *Am J Clin Nutr* 30, no. 2 (1977): 160–70.

Loma Linda University. "New Loma Linda University Study Underscores Value of Nutrient-Dense Walnuts in Weight Management." Life Extension Foundation, *LEF Daily News*: Business Wire, December 16, 2005. http://www.lef.org/news/LefDailyNews.htm?NewsID=3088&Section=NUTRITION.

Medical College of Wisconsin. "Very High Fiber Diet Lowers Blood Glucose in Diabetics." *HealthLink.* http://healthlink.mcw.edu/article/958073584.html.

Netter, Frank H. *The CIBA Collection of Medical Illustrations.* Vol. 3, *Digestive System*, Part III: *Liver, Biliary Tract and Pancreas.* 2nd ed. New York: CIBA Pharmaceutical, 1972.

————. *The CIBA Collection of Medical Illustrations.* Vol. 4, *Endocrine System and Selected Metabolic Diseases.* New York: CIBA Pharmaceutical, 1970.

Nicklas, Barbara, ed. *Endurance Exercise and Adipose Tissue.* Boca Raton, FL: CRC Press, 2002.

Research Consortium Sustainable Animal Production. "Animal Nutrition: Resources and New Challenges: Summary." http://agriculture.de/acms1/conf6/ws8sum.htm.

Schuenke, Mark D., Richard P. Mikat, and Jeffrey M. McBride. "Effect of an Acute Period of Resistance Exercise on Excess Post-Exercise Oxygen Consumption: Implications for Body Mass Management." *Eur J Appl Physiol* 86, no. 5 (2002): 411–17.

Shomon, Mary J. *Living Well with Hypothyroidism: What Your Doctor Doesn't Tell You . . . That You Need to Know.* New York: Avon Books, 2000.

Stitt, Paul A. *Beating the Food Giants.* Manitowoc, WI: Natural Press, 1993.

University of Wisconsin. "Endocrine Disrupters: Crossed Wires? EPA Tackles Hormone Disrupters." *The Why Files.* http://whyfiles.org/045env_hormone/main1.html.

U.S. Dept. of Health and Human Services and U.S. Environmental Protection Agency. "What You Need to Know About Mercury in Fish and Shellfish: 2004 EPA and FDA Advice for Women Who Might Become Pregnant, Women Who Are Pregnant, Nursing Mothers, Young Children." EPA-823-R-04-005, March 2004. http://www.cfsan.fda.gov/~dms/admehg3.html.

U.S. EPA (U.S. Environmental Protection Agency). "Endocrine Disruptors Research Initiative." http://www.epa.gov/endocrine/.

Walnut Marketing Board. "Further Proof: Walnuts Protective for People with Type 2 Diabetes." *PressRoom*, July 6, 2005. http://www.walnuts.org/inthenews/pressroom.php.

————. "New Study Shows Melatonin in Walnuts Protective Against Cancer and Heart Disease." *Press Room*, September 13, 2005. http://www.walnuts.org/inthenews/pressroom.php.

Yancy, William S., Jr., Maren K. Olsen, John R. Guyton, Ronna P. Bakst, and Eric C. Westman. "A Low-Carbohydrate, Ketogenic Diet versus a Low-Fat Diet to Treat Obesity and Hyperlipidemia." *Ann Intern Med* 140, no. 10 (2004): 769–77.

Resources

Dr. Berg's Heal*thy*Self Tip of the Week

If you would like to receive my free Heal*thy*Self tips of the week, go to http://www.bergdiets.com/ and sign up.

The 7 Principles of Fat Burning

To recommend *The 7 Principles of Fat Burning* to a friend, have them go to http://www.bergdiets.com/. This site shows a video of Dr. Berg covering the four body types, and they can also take a free Body Type Quiz.

Acupressure Stress Elimination Technique

For more information on Dr. Berg's acupressure technique and to locate a certified practitioner near you, go to http://www.drbergacupressure.com/.

Weight Loss Support

With our Internet Fat-Burning-Tracker Coach, the exact program can be tailor-made to your body type. To find a health coach in your area, go to http://www.fbtcoach.com/.

E-mail Hotline

While doing the program, if you need to clarify a point or have a question for which you cannot find the answer in this book, you may send your query to our e-mail hotline service: quickquestion@bergdiets.com.

CraveStopper

If you crave sugar during stressful times and need that extra support, order a bottle of CraveStopper by going to http://www.bergdiets.com/.

Organic Cruciferous Food & Organic Cruciferous Sprouts Food

You can order these products from the Health & Wellness Center by calling 800-816-8184 during normal business hours or by going online to http://www.bergdiets.com/. Each bottle contains 250 tablets and costs $36.00.

Bran Crispbread

http://www.brancrispbread.com/

Cranberry Juice Powder

http://www.usjuice.com/
Click on "Unsweetened Cranberry Powder."

Enzymes to Help with Digestion

If you have a sensitivity to certain vegetables or beans and get uncomfortable bloating, you can order these specific enzymes from this website: http://www.bean-zyme.com/.

Exercise Monitoring Device

This unit is a nondiagnostic educational tool to help you monitor your own exercise. It is an excellent method for finding out your personalized recovery periods between exercise bouts, making an exercise program very individualized and more effective. For further information, go to http://www.bergdiets.com/.

Ezekiel Sprouted Grain Products

http://www.foodforlife.com/

Mochi

http://www.grainaissance.com/

Standard Process Inc.

The Standard Process purification and weight management programs include four excellent products—SP Green Food, SP Complete, SP Cleanse and Gastro-Fiber—which can be used in place of Organic Cruciferous Food. Standard Process provides concentrated food complexes, and I have been using them in my clinic for over a decade. However, you have to obtain these supplements through a healthcare practitioner. To find a practitioner who uses Standard Process products, you can call the company at 800-848-5061 (USA) or go to their website at http://www.standardprocess.com/.

The Future of Food Video

http://www.thefutureoffood.com/

Index

Page numbers in italics refer to charts or illustrations.

Fat-Burning Tracker Web Support

Benefits

- Weekly graph to see how close you are to fat-burning mode based on food and exercise input.

- Nine bar graphs on food-hormone triggers to isolate hidden sources of weight gain, both water weight and actual fat.

- Five graphs on energy, sleep, digestion, cravings and stress levels, to see how these graphs correlate to weight and inches lost.

- Sodium – potassium ratio graph— important for fluid weight.

- Exercise graphs to identify whether you are maximizing fat burning, based on your body type for both aerobic and anaerobic.

- Get tailor-made recommendations on what you need to do to maximize fat burning.

- Graph your omega 3 and omega 6 fatty acid ratios to make sure they are in range.

- Dialog with your health coach and get answers to your specific questions.

  And much, much more . . .

Go to www.fbtcoach.com.

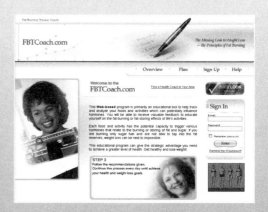

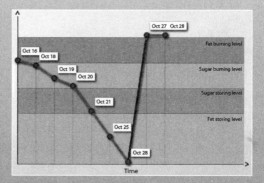

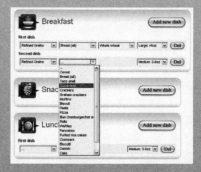

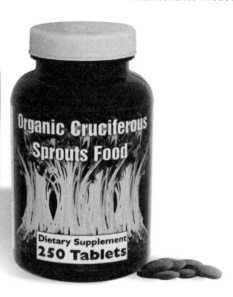

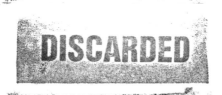